Warning

You are about to get a heavy dose of commonsense methods that could virtually erase **Alzheimer's Disease** from the future of our children, delay its onset for senior citizens, and help those with **AD** to enjoy a better quality of life.

Published by UCS PRESS

UCS PRESS is an imprint of MarJim Books
PO Box 13025
Tucson, AZ 85732-3025

Copyright © 2011 by James F. Watson

Cover design by Marty Dobkins

ISBN 978-0-943247-30-6

Author's Note

Common sense is a commodity that is in very short supply these days. How else can you explain our society's deterioration? No longer is job stability the norm in our lives. And to many even the roofs over their heads are in jeopardy, as their home values plummet and thoughts of foreclosure torment their minds. Indebtedness is becoming the norm, as savings dwindle, as we struggle just to get by. And now calm, once the norm, is being replaced with stress. Childhood diseases that were once rare are increasing each year, and many adults are spending more time with their doctors than with there own families, as family units break down. General good health is becoming a thing of the past.

The paradox is that we live in a society where money for health care and medical research is at an all-time high. Some statistics claim 17% of our economy is based around health care. You would think that things would be getting better instead of worse.

Where is the common sense in it all?

I am just old enough to remember a world where the majority of people were kind, compassionate, and trustworthy with one's word being confirmed with a handshake. And once given, that word was rarely broken.

That was a world that had consistency. The vast majority of children still were growing up in family units in which the members cared about each other.

It was a world that I dearly miss.

Looking back to my childhood I don't recall even knowing the term Alzheimer's Disease. AD wasn't nearly as prevalent as it is today. Over 5,000,000 adults are confirmed AD victims with many others not yet aware that they have AD. What is frightening is that millions more in North America will be diagnosed as having AD just a few years into this new century.

These AD statistics should be lower. And they could be lower, a lot lower.

But how can this be achieved?

The answer, I believe, is to be found in commonsense approaches that will be presented in this book.

It is true that millions of dollars are being spent annually on AD research in the United States and in other countries. But how many of those dollars are going into the search for preventive means to stop AD from occurring in the first place? How many of those dollars will lead to the development of new drugs that will make billions of more dollars for major drug companies?

Why would multi-billion-dollar corporations jeopardize their profits by funding research to find, God forbid, a cure for a cash cow disease? If the research will not lead to a drug that can be patented, you can bet your sweet bippy it will be dropped.

If there is a way to prevent the onset of a disease, I want to know what that way is.

If a loved one or I already had that disease, I would want to know what could be done to minimize its effects.

In either case I would want to know if the goal is achievable by minimal drug taking or possibly by natural means alone.

Up front I confess that I am not associated with any medical school, major research laboratory, foundation, or major corporation. I am not a physician or a psychologist, but a self-taught neuroscientist and concerned citizen who has discovered commonsense means of dealing with and preventing AD. In this book I present those means to you in as unbiased a manner as I possibly can.

There is research that could be done to prove my beliefs. Although this book is not the result of any profit motive, it would be fantastic should this book get into enough people's hands so that the research could be done by LODGE Creek Research Center. LODGE would stand for "Locating the Origin of Disease through Genetics and Environment."

There is so much I have learned in the field of environmental stimulants that I want to pass on to you and others. Much of that knowledge is incorporated in this book. My hope is that you will find on these pages the answers to questions you have about AD.

James F. Watson

Dedication

To Mom and Dad for being so special and always being there for me. And especially to Dad's memory...he died the day the book manuscript was completed.

Acknowledgment

Eternal thanks go to my wife Sandra, sons James, Michael and Noah; and Brittany, whom we wanted so much to adopt. You've all shown me how important it is to receive unconditional love on an ongoing basis.

Table of Contents

Introduction

Like most individuals it took a tragic event to open my eyes and truly examine the world around me. The tragic event of slowly losing the one I hold most dear to my heart, my wife Sandy. After 20 years of a most enjoyable relationship our lives together started to fall apart. Compassion was replaced with conscientiousness, calm with anger, trust with distrust, pleasure with stress, depression had set in and good health was a thing of the past. No longer did Sandy awaken each morning with the zest for life she once had. What seamed like overnight our world together just fell apart, with no clear explanation in sight.

Where had it all gone? And most bewildering to myself, was the fact we had just come full circle in the game of life. We had just completed the task of raising two children with much success, with little difficulties along the way. We were financially stable with retirement in sight and nearing the completion of our dream home. At the young age of 39 we had it all, including a second home on the water to retreat to.

Over the years our main goal was to fulfill the needs of our children first, Sandy as a stay home mom, dabbling with a few jobs along the way when times got tough, and me as the principle provider. Our objectives were simple: fulfill our children's dreams while they are young, as we only get one chance to do it right so they will reward our efforts in the future. We placed our goals on hold, figuring that soon the time will come to fulfill our own as our children leave the nest to create lives of their own.

Well, that time had come. I was very focused on the future and looking forward to shifting our needs back to each other like we had in the past when we first meet. You know, the first time you truly fall in love and nothing else matters except just being together and fulfilling each other's needs?

But somewhere along the way Sandy had completely derailed; not focusing on the future but on the perils of the past, with much fear of the new life she was about to enter.

What had happened, where had it all gone, and what was I to do? Never before have I seen such a rapid reversal of one's personality.

As time went on things only worsened. Sandy's compassion for life was gone, arguing was the norm, defense shields were built, and the pleasures of life were nonexistent.

From expert to expert we went, with diagnoses ranging from menopause, to depression, to just general low self-esteem, unhappy marriage (due to us wanting to live the traditional ways in an untraditional society) and possibly a thyroid problem. There were so many diagnoses with the same symptoms.

Each day brought new problems: balancing a checkbook became a thing of the past, socializing with others was completely out of the question, and her short-term memory was slipping away. The first signs of Alzheimer's were showing up.

With now something to focus on, it was time to take action and confront the matter most people would prefer to ignore or pass on to others. Early in my research I was astonished that AD – once a rare disease – had become quite common. It is no longer a disease affecting just the elderly population; individuals of all ages show full-blown symptoms of AD.

Why has this happened?

Even more tragic, why was there no cure?

There were only drugs to possibly delay its further onset by six or so months, no true research as to the cause of AD, and very little research in the field of prevention. There was, and continues to be, only massive amounts of research in the field of genetics and new drugs.

With few answers in sight, I decided to take charge. Like I had done in business, I took the commonsense approach, and concentrated on the successes of others instead of their failures. What was so different in their lives than in Sandy's? What factors helped them to age with grace? Why had a once rare disease now become so common? What was its cause?

From the day my first son was born, I have dabbled in trying to understand the mind. Why, after years of trying to quit smoking, did it become so simple for me to do? And why was my grandfather able to simply abandon a drinking habit upon the birth of his first grandchild?

The stimulants around you that control your mind are very powerful. I plunged into heavy research. What external stimulants – or lack of – were taking Sandy down the path of AD? Soon hours turned into days, and days into years. I discovered AD's many causes; also, unconscious methods to prevent AD used by those who age with grace.

Through applying these methods, Sandy is improving. I believe she is about seventy-five percent back. The other twenty-five percent should soon return.

Helping her fully recover is truly my "magnificent obsession."

James F. Watson

"With Alzheimer's people, there's no such thing as having a day which is like another day. Every day is separate…it's as if every day you have never seen anything before like what you're seeing right now."

Cary Henderson
AD victim, while still able to dictate his thoughts on a tape recorder.

Chapter 1: The Great Mind Robber

The title of this chapter is a good answer to the question, "What is Alzheimer's Disease?"

It is an important question that has ramifications for a hefty chunk of the United States population. In 1996 there were an estimated four million-plus Alzheimer's victims in the U.S. That number has since grown to over five million. When you consider that for each person suffering from Alzheimer's Disease (AD) there are at least eight other persons affected, be it spouse, children, relatives, or close friends, the number of people directly influenced by AD is about forty-five million.

And the statistics just keep getting worse. If it were an infectious disease, it would be declared a plague and one-sixth of the U.S. population would be quarantined in an effort to halt its spread. Projections are that fourteen to fifteen million Americans will have contracted AD by mid-century. That is a tripling of victims in only fifty years!

Over ten percent of adults at age 65 have AD; nearly fifty percent aged 85 or older. But most people already know that your odds of getting AD greatly increase as you get older; however, did you know that more and more people are being diagnosed as having AD while still in their 40's and 50's? In another chapter I will share with you a case involving several women in their 30's who are showing classic AD symptoms.

From rare disease to mass killer

In less than a century, AD has gone from being considered a rare disease to one of the leading causes of death among American adults. Half of all nursing home patients are believed to have AD.

Dr. Alois Alzheimer (1864-1915), a German physician, made a presentation of medical findings at a meeting in 1907. He discussed the case of a 51-year-old woman whose "symptoms included depression, hallucinations, and dementia." He had performed an autopsy and was startled to find a great decrease of cells in the cerebral cortex and "clumps of filaments between the nerve cells."

Neither Dr. Alzheimer nor any of the other participants at that meeting had ever seen anything like what the autopsy revealed. They only knew that it was a debilitating, progressive disease. Dr. Alzheimer identified the disease, which soon bore his name, but he had no idea as to cause, treatment, cure, or prevention.

Were Dr. Alzheimer alive today, I believe that he would be appalled at the statistics. And he'd probably be absolutely aghast at the cash cow AD has become for the medical and drug industries. "Why do so many people have this disease?" he would ask. "I just don't get it. Isn't anybody doing anything about it?"

Frankly, what's mainly being done is research that focuses on creating new drugs, or methods of manipulating genes, or implanting cells. Fancy-sounding stuff, to be sure, but very little research is being done on cause which could lead to prevention, and that is where my main focus lies.

There are nearly three million caregivers out there and many millions of family members looking for answers. And they are all tired of hearing about new discoveries only to be told, "We will get back with you in five or ten years after we study it."

What ever happened to common sense?

If it isn't spelled "common cents" and can't quickly be compounded into huge bottom lines, the big drug companies and other industry giants who back most of the medical research that is done today just hit the ignore button and merrily go on their profit-making way. Supporting evidence of the truth of this statement will be presented in other chapters.

Common sense is what this book is about. That's the path I've chosen to follow as an independent investigator and researcher. It certainly is the "road less traveled."

Seven decades later

It was not until the 1980's that neuroscientists – folks who study the brain – began to figure out what the "clumps of filaments between the nerve cells" actually are.

When Dr. Alzheimer did the now famous biopsy, he found dense deposits outside and around the nerve cells in the woman's brain. Inside the cells were twisted strands of fiber. Such dense deposits are today called neuritic plaques while the twisted strands of fiber are known as neurofibrillary tangles. Neuroscientists then discovered the proteins that comprise the plaques and tangles. We'll discuss this later. Don't worry; we won't get into a discourse of ten-dollar words. I just mentioned the plaques and tangles here as a way of showing that it took about seventy years before AD research really got out of first gear.

However, there was a major scientific discovery in the mid-1970's involving an important neurotransmitter that will be covered in Chapter Two.

Ten warning signs of Alzheimer's Disease

The Alzheimer's Association has developed a checklist of common AD symptoms. (Some of the symptoms are common with other dementing illnesses.) If the individual you are concerned about displays several of these symptoms get that person to a doctor with a track record of knowing how to diagnose AD.

Memory loss that affects job skills

It's normal to occasionally forget assignments, colleagues' names or a business associate's telephone number and remember them later. Those with a dementia, such as AD, may forget things more often, and not remember them later.

Difficulty performing familiar tasks

Busy people can be so distracted from time to time that they may leave the carrots on the stove and only remember to serve them at the end of the meal. People with AD could prepare a meal and not only forget to serve it, but forget they made it.

Problems with language

Everyone has trouble finding the right word at times, but a person with AD might forget simple words or substitute inappropriate words, making his or her sentence incomprehensible.

Disorientation of time and place

It's normal to forget the day of the week or your destination for a moment. But people with AD can become lost on their own street, not knowing where they are, how they got there, or how to get back home.

Poor or decreased judgment

People can become so immersed in an activity that they temporarily forget the child they're watching. People with AD could forget entirely the child under their care. They might also dress inappropriately, wearing several shirts or blouses.

Problems with abstract thinking

Balancing a checkbook might be disconcerting when the task is more complicated than usual. Someone with AD could forget completely what the numbers are and what needs to be done with them.

Misplacing things

Anyone can temporarily misplace a wallet or keys. A person with AD might put things in inappropriate places: an iron in the freezer; a wristwatch in the sugar bowl.

Changes in mood or behavior

Everyone becomes sad or moody from time to time. Someone with AD can exhibit rapid mood swings – from calm to tears to anger – for no apparent reason.

Changes in personality

People's personalities ordinarily change somewhat with age. But a person with AD can change drastically, becoming extremely confused, suspicious, or fearful.

Loss of initiative

It's normal to tire of housework, business activities, or social obligations, but most people regain their initiative. The person with AD might become very passive and require cues and prompting to become involved.

How is AD diagnosed?

There is no single diagnostic test. AD is diagnosed by first ruling out other diseases and illnesses that can cause dementia. Whether conducted by your family physician or a team of specialists, the process usually involves the following:

A thorough medical history of the person with symptoms of AD as well as family members.

An assessment of the person's mental status.

A thorough physical exam.

A neurological exam.

A series of lab tests.

Psychological and other exams.

A diagnosis obtained in this manner is considered to be 80 to 90 percent accurate. Even today, the only 100 percent way to confirm that a person had AD is through an autopsy.

AD has three basic stages

While researchers have come up with different scales to measure the progression of AD, usually citing ranges of five to seven stages, experienced caregivers consider AD to have three phases: mild, moderate, and severe. As the progression of symptoms varies from person to person, there can be some overlapping of these symptoms; however, this is a pretty good outline overview.

Mild Symptoms

Conscientiousness which declines
Vulnerability to stress which increases
Occasional depression
Loss of sense of smell

Moderate Symptoms

Confusion and memory loss
Disorientation; getting lost in familiar surroundings
Problems with routine tasks
Changes in personality and judgment

Severe Symptoms

Loss of speech
Loss of appetite; weight loss
Loss of bladder and bowel control
Total dependence on caregiver

How long AD victims live after diagnosis varies greatly. Some live just a few years more while others may live another twenty years or so. The one constant is that watching a loved one suffering from AD is a sad experience. It's like viewing a crime being committed in slow motion. You see it happening and yet you feel utterly helpless in being able to do anything about it. All the while you sense that your loved one's mind is slowly being stolen. Which, in a sense, is exactly what is happening.

You can play an important part in the fight to stop this Great Mind Robber.

How, you ask?

You can do it by participating in the questionnaire included in the last chapter of this book. With massive numbers of people answering the one hundred questions, and doing it anonymously, the results will lead to a better understanding of possible causes of AD and, therefore, help lead to means of slowing down AD and eventually preventing its onslaught.

Chapter One: Key Points to Remember

AD has rapidly become one of the leading causes of death among American adults.

One-half of all nursing home patients are believed to have AD.

Only within the past 20 years have scientists figured out what the "clumps of filaments between the nerve cells" are that Dr. Alzheimer discovered nearly 100 years ago.

You can help in the fight to stop AD by participating in the questionnaire presented in Chapter Nineteen.

"If we knew what it was we were doing, it would not be called research, would it?"

Albert Einstein

Chapter 2: What causes Alzheimer's?

Trying to pinpoint a primary cause of AD is like trying to see wind. You know it's there because you can see the effects like swaying trees and rolling tumbleweeds; but no matter how hard you try you just cannot see the wind.

Scientists and caregivers know only too well what the effects of AD are. They just have not been able to figure out what causes AD.

Is there really a primary cause of AD?

Or is it possible that there are multiple, perhaps even many causes?

And, if there are indeed many causes, could at least some of these causes be unmasked through a commonsense research approach?

An overview of AD and the brain

Before we get into a discussion of causes, it would be good to briefly go over what scientists have verified about AD activity in the brain.

AD begins in the entorhinal cortex and goes from there to the hippocampus, a way station important in memory formation. Over time it gradually spreads to other regions, particularly the cerebral cortex, the outer area of the brain that is involved in functions such as language and reason.

In the areas attacked by AD the nerve cells (neurons) degenerate, losing their connections (synapses) with other neurons. The result is that neurons begin to die.

When hippocampal neurons degenerate short-term memory begins to fail. Also, the ability to do routine tasks starts to deteriorate. As AD advances through the cerebral cortex the ability to use language properly becomes harder and harder to do. Frustrations of all kinds beset the victim. With the progression of AD often come disturbing behaviors such as wandering and agitation. In its ruthless onslaught AD eventually erases one's ability to recognize even close family members or to communicate in any way. Finally all sense of self worth seems to vanish and the victim becomes totally dependent on others for care.

It really is a heart-breaking, gut-wrenching experience to see a loved one go through such a devastating transformation. My wife's grandmother went through it. And, as I said in the Introduction, my initial focus on AD research is to do everything I can to help my wife avoid the same fate.

I sincerely believe that the early stages of AD can be reversed. We will discuss that later. Now on to our discussion of possible causes.

Like looking for needles in haystacks

There are hundreds of billions of neurons in the brain. Any one of them can have thousands, even hundreds of thousands, of connections with other neurons. Chemical messengers, such as neurotransmitters, hormones, and growth factors, travel along the myriads of neuron branches. They link each neuron with others in an unbelievably complex communications network.

Scientists believe that somewhere in this massive signaling system lies the cause of AD. This train of thought began in the mid-1970s with the discovery that levels of a neurotransmitter called acetylcholine fell sharply in people with AD. It was an important discovery for at least three reasons:

Acetycholine is a vital neurotransmitter in the process of forming memories.

It is the neurotransmitter commonly used by neurons in the hippocampus and cerebral cortex, areas that are devastated by AD.

It linked AD with biochemical changes in the brain.

Acetycholine became and continues to be the focus of many studies. Its levels fall some during the normal aging process; however, it drops by about ninety percent in victims of AD. Evidence links this decline to memory impairment. Scientists have looked for ways to boost its levels as a possible treatment for AD.

Other neurotransmitters such as serotonin, somatostatin, and noradrenaline have been found to be at lower than normal levels in those with AD.

I could go on, expanding this discussion into what happens when a message carried by a neurotransmitter has crossed the synapse, what part receptors play, phospholid abnormalities, beta amyloid, but it really is not necessary (Although in another chapter we will discuss beta amyloid and how to combat it.). Meanwhile, you get the idea A-OK that scientists are concentrating their research efforts on what goes on inside the brain. Their findings go toward development of drugs and gene manipulation but contribute little to cause discovery.

Which is where I come in. To me, the questions that more and more researchers should be asking are these:

What if there are things that happen outside the brain that are the real triggers for what takes place inside the brain?

If so, what might these external causes be?

Job security is one reason why few researchers take such a commonsense approach. Were they to start finding answers to these questions, the need for more drugs would decrease, research funding from major drug companies would be cut off, and their jobs would go bye-bye.

First, take a look at changes in our society

Look at the world around you. What do you see? Do you see the same things that your parents saw? And do you think that they saw the same things that their parents (your grandparents) saw?

Now mentally step out of yourself and look closely at this representation of three generations.

Which generation's world had the strongest emphasis on family?

In which generation did marriage vows have the most meaning?

At what point in which generation did divorce seem to become rampant?

And in which generation did the institution of family itself come under attack in seemingly every aspect of life?

What about such general categories as moral values and judgments, political correctness, even respect for public figures?

Which generation felt the most secure as to terms of self-worth and overall physical safety, be it at home, in school, or out in a public setting?

Do you think any of these generations looked or seems to look like it is falling apart at the seams?

Point blank: We live in the one generation that is the most fraught with change of the greatest magnitude of perhaps any previous generation, definitely since the first generation after closure of the Dark Ages. Indeed, we live in a generation of uncertainties. And the things that are certain give us an even greater feeling of uncertainty about our futures. It is certain that more and more companies and industries will down size. Acts of violence in our country and other countries around the world will continue to increase. Fewer medical and other benefits will be provided for employees.

Greater numbers of children are growing up in our society really knowing at best only one natural parent. Even then most of these children will see more of baby sitters and other care providers, including school teachers, than they will of that one parent.

Now just what does all this have to do with Alzheimer's?

A lot if you look closely enough at generational changes. For example, is it coincidence that the rapid increase in the number of people with AD has mirrored the pace at which the break-up of the family structure has occurred? Or that it is rising in proportion to the increase of myriads of stress factors in our society?

Common sense, then, indicates the need to consider a wide variety of external influences that might contribute to one's showing the outward signs of AD later in life.

Low emotional stimulation

It is my contention that the greatest underlying factor in AD is a person's history and its continued effect on a person's life. That means total history right from the moment of birth.

Babies that do not receive consistent, positive emotional stimulation are given a handicap that might not be overcome the rest of their lives. If there is not a large amount of such stimulation, the networks of neurons that are created in the brain will be smaller than they could or should be.

Tremendous foundational networks are formed during the weeks and months after birth. The brain is setting itself up to function in a particular manner for the rest of that person's life. Loving parents and caregivers can provide the stimulation needed to help the brain set up what later on might become defense systems against AD.

Although these networks are one of the most important factors in the onset of AD, I am not aware of any research being done that considers such networks to be primary factors. That is an oversight that I believe needs to be rectified.

Too many changes of emotional stimulants

When AD was rare, most persons' environmental and emotional stimuli were quite consistent. Family units remained together usually in the same communities. Friend-ships were limited, often lasting a lifetime, and jobs, whether stressful or pleasurable, were retained for many years.

Life was pretty repetitive. Through such repetitiveness neurons containing memory received constant impulses that, in a sense, kept those neurons healthy. That in turn prevented cells from degenerating due to lack of what neuroscientists call excitement.

In today's society, especially over the past three decades, environmental and emotional stimuli have become quite sporadic. Intact family units, if not already, are fast becoming the exception to the norm. Friendships and intimate relationships with many individuals on a short-term basis are common, as are job and career changes.

The result is that many more neurons are excited thereby creating many more connections. The problem is that a lot of these neurons and connections are never going to be excited on a consistent basis through life. The networks are thereby weakened, making the neurons very susceptible to gene mutation from lack of cell nutrition. Eventually the cells program themselves for suicide through a process known as apopotosis. Once enough cells are dead, AD can develop. Later in this book we'll discuss ways of delaying and possibly preventing this process from taking place.

Abrupt stimuli changes can trigger problems

An abrupt change in stimuli means an abrupt change in the production and secretion of hormones and other chemicals that are necessary to sustain many bodily functions. Two good examples of such change are retirement and the loss of a loving spouse.

When one retires stimulation of massive neuron networks decreases and so does the production of hormones. As these large networks begin to break up one will become vulnerable to the onset of AD. Beta amyloid plaques eventually will start to form and the immune system will face an attack that it cannot withstand.

Over the life of a marriage, especially if it is a long one, very large networks are formed of both pleasure and painful experiences. Especially in cases where the surviving spouse had depended almost solely on his or her mate for stimulation, the abrupt change leads to a rapid weakening of the immune system.

We will provide tools that can be used to reinforce one's immune system in the wake of retirement or death of a spouse.

Poor diet can lead to road of no return

Let's expand that old saw from "You are what you eat" to "You are what you eat and drink." I say this because diet includes not only the food we intake but also the liquids that we consume.

An imbalanced diet, especially from early childhood, will set one up for many disease possibilities, including AD. If one receives poor nutrition as a child that person usually receives poor stimulation of the mind. The mind needs proteins to help its many areas function properly. And that is one need that has been drastically under-met over the past thirty years. Balance is the key word. We will discuss diet effects pertaining to children in the next chapter. An extensive diet discussion is in a chapter later in this book.

Environmental factors

Of growing concern are the many herbicides/pesticides that contain carbamates or organophosphates or both. These toxic chemicals inhibit cholinesterase, which is a necessary enzyme in the blood. Exposure can lead to disrupted muscle coordination.

Be careful using products that contain Ronnel, Malathion, Diazion, Dursban, and Parathion. They are found as main ingredients in many over-the-counter preparations used to kill unwanted weeds on driveways, patios, and lawns.

It is increasingly possible to become exposed to dangerous chemicals simply by living near a plant or industrial complex where toxic chemicals are used in various processes. Put it this way: if all the fish die in your neighborhood pond or lake, and there is a plant nearby, would you keep on drinking the tap water?

The growing case against aluminum

Despite the fact that autopsies have shown an over-abundance of aluminum in the brains of AD victims, there are still some researchers who contend there is no proof that aluminum has any bearing at all as an AD-causing factor.

Could this possibly be a result of the aluminum industry providing extensive funding for research in areas of gene manipulation and gene-splicing?

And could an ulterior motive for funding the research be to draw attention away from aluminum itself as being a possible cause of AD?

Aluminum seems to be everywhere. In toothpaste tubes, deodorant, soft drink cans, cookware, consumer drugs, antacids, aspirin, and many other products. It contaminates drinking water and milk.

Complex ionic aluminosilicates (aluminum compounds) go directly to the brain through the olfactory system. Is it a coincidence that much of the damage typical of AD is found in the olfactory regions of the brain?

Aluminosilicates are found in dust from talcum powder, baby powder, cat-box litter, cement, asphalt mixes, tobacco smoke, and ashes.

The tobacco industry is being hit by multi-million-dollar lawsuits as a result of massive deaths caused by long-term smoking habits. Some people believe that the aluminum industry might be next on the lawsuit chopping block.

Then there's the fluoride reign of terror

The aluminum by-product fluoride affects our lives via toothpaste, water supplies, and other products. Many tests in various countries have repeatedly confirmed the dangerous toxicity of fluoride (fluorine).

Yet in the United States most of the municipal water supplies are fluoride treated. A dramatic result is a more widespread and rapid decrease in the efficiency of the immune systems of populations that drink fluoridated water. Dentists brainwash parents into thinking that fluoride treatments will help strengthen the teeth of their children and decrease the odds of tooth decay.

You know what? The truth has been brought out in many tests that show exactly the opposite. For example, a study of 400,000 Indian schoolchildren from 1973-1993 showed that the higher the fluoride concentration in the water, the more cavities occurred.

But it's not the cavity arena that is so scary. What fluoride does to the brain is reason enough to eliminate contact between humans and fluoride in as many ways as possible and as quickly as possible.

Here are a few of the proven toxic affects of fluoride:

Destroys about sixty enzymes including cytochrome C and cholinesterase that handle oxygen.

Causes genetic change in sperm and other cells.

Leads to an increase in Downs Syndrome of 250 percent with 70 percent of those developing cataracts.

Increases the rate of infant mortality, spontaneous abortions, and miscarriages.

Increases the rate of infant birth defects.

Let's hope that efforts soon succeed in bringing a stop to the use and spread of this deadly destroyer. Meanwhile, avoid anything that has been fluoridated or has fluorine in it like the plague.

Could memory suppression be a possible cause?

One of my theories is that the suppression of memories over a long period of time can contribute to the onset of AD. There has been at least one test that I am aware of that seems to support my contention.

The test involved several groups of women undergraduates who were asked to view slides of men with various degrees of obvious physical injuries. Half of the women were asked to hide any feelings of emotion by maintaining what gamblers call a "poker face."

After the slide show a surprise memory-recall test was given to all participants. The women who had been asked to suppress their emotions scored collectively lower on the exam.

If short-term memory was affected by such a brief test just think what affect memory suppression over many years might have on the brain? You would be causing neuron networks to basically die of excitement starvation. Those neglected neurons would eventually start dying and AD symptoms would follow.

Stress might play a big causative role

Actually, it is not so much the stress itself as it is how a person deals with that stress that determines whether the odds of getting AD go up or down. We'll discuss ways of dealing with stress in another chapter.

The negative consequences of stress are for real. When facing what our brain perceives as a stressful situation, be it a final exam or a dreaded job review, the brain prepares one for what is known as the "fight or flight" response. The chemical cortisol is produced as dramatic metabolic changes occur throughout one's body.

Should the situation pass and one has not fought or taken flight, the cortisol has not been counteracted and sticks around to do damage. Build-ups of cortisol attack the immune system and result in the slaughter of neurons responsible for memory. Gaps start appearing in short-term memory networks. As more neurons die AD becomes more of a possibility.

What about "sugarless" products?

Greed, pure and simple, has led to an avalanche of products that contain sweetening substances that I am absolutely convinced are already in the process of assuring that millions more of our population will be ravaged by AD.

When several young women still in their thirties began showing AD symptoms, a search was made to see what factor might show up in their case studies. The only truly common factor was that each of the women was a diet drinkaholic. They were guzzling aluminum can after aluminum can of soft drinks sweetened by aspartame.

Aspartame is the technical name for the brand names, NutraSweet, Equal, Spoonful, and EqualMeasure. It is comprised of three chemicals: Aspartic acid, phenylalanine, and methanol. The book, *Prescription for Nutritional Healing,* by James and Phyllis Balch, lists aspartame under the category of "chemical poison."

Methanol, also known as wood alcohol, converts to formaldehyde in beverages that are heated to over 86 degrees F.

Hundreds of thousands of diet soft drinks were consumed by our armed forces personnel during Desert Shield and Desert Storm, often in desert settings with temperatures soaring to the 120-degree range. Is there any wonder that so many of them returned home with numerous disorders similar to what has been documented in persons who have been chemically poisoned by formaldehyde?

Think about it. You don't have to have the mind of a rocket scientist to figure out that aspartame is poison. The proof is on the table. Be safe and run from any product that says "sugarless." That is one of the best AD prevention measures you can take.

Markers or risk factors

There are a number of what researchers call markers or risk factors while stopping short of claiming that they are causes of AD. Included are history of seizures, poor language and writing ability, exposure to excessive amounts of zinc or lead, low educational level, head injuries, and calcium build-ups in the brain.

It is probably a very safe conclusion to say that a number of factors can lead to the onset of AD. However, the trigger that sets one person on the path toward AD might not be the same trigger that propels another person in that direction. Having a good general knowledge of the possibilities will give you a basis for forming a plan of prevention or a plan of treatment, depending upon your situation or needs.

Chapter Two: Key points to remember

There are many factors that can lead to one having AD later in life.

Knowing one's life history is important in discovering how to prevent AD.

Social changes are factors.

As are:
Low emotional stimulation
Too many changes of emotional stimulants
Abrupt stimuli changes
Poor diet
Environmental influences such as herbicides and pesticides.
Aluminum, especially its by-product fluoride (fluorine)
Memory suppression
How one deals with stress
Aspartame, which is a "chemical poison"

You're encouraged to take The Alzheimer's Self-Test

I thought the best place to put this vitally informative test was between Chapters Two and Three. By taking this test, you will gain a good idea of the possibility that you will avoid or become a victim of Alzheimer's Disease.

Remember, once a rare disease, Alzheimer's has become the 4th leading cause of death. In 1996 there were an estimated four million-plus Alzheimer's victims in the U.S. That number has since grown to over five million, with predictions that these statistics are going to rise to fifteen million by the year 2050 as the baby boomers age.

Are you interested in becoming one of these statistics, as your mind takes the progressive path back to childhood? Or are you ready to take control now while your mind is still intact and enjoy those retirement years with your spouse and others?

Decisions, decisions…make them while you can, because soon others might be making them for you.

Having many causes, AD has become a most difficult disease to diagnose, treat or prevent. With a definite diagnoses only confirmed upon autopsy, you must ask yourself, is it truly AD, a disease that has no cure, or just one of the many forms of dementia so common today? At which point does a reversible dementia turn into full-blown AD, a now non-reversible disease?

Upon the onset or diagnosis of other diseases you have the cognitive capacity to think for yourself in choosing a treatment plan or a reasonable lifestyle change in reversing its onset. This is not so true with AD. There are so many factors you must consider at a most vulnerable time, as your mind starts slipping away.

With AD, time is of the essence. As with each passing day you further lose your cognitive capacity to take action against its further onset. Consider the progress of AD. It very much mimics the reversal of the mind back to childhood: a period in your life where reasonable decisions were most difficult and usually made by others for you.

Are you ready to take that path...or do you want to take control now?

Taking control at the first signs of AD is essential, before it starts taking control over you. Do not take the path of denial so many take out of fear. Fear that soon you will be headed down the path of a non-reversible disease with no cure, accompanied by a long, drawn-out death of anywhere from 8 to 20 years. Taking control over your denial is the first step to a full recovery. Fully evaluate the situation while your mind is still pretty much there to assist you. As with each passing day it's going to become more difficult as dementia sets in. With its multiple causes, who better qualified than yourself in evaluating your past, in discovering what is leading you down the path of dementia and then eventually Alzheimer's? Only by evaluating your life from conception till the present are you going to find the answers. Below are the many known factors that both help cause and prevent Alzheimer's. Step up and take the test. Evaluate your life to learn how vulnerable each and every one of us is to Alzheimer's.

Childhood

The first step in understanding your vulnerability to AD begins by evaluating your childhood. From conception to birth there are many factors that determine brain size, including mother's nutrition, general health, age, drug use (caffeine, alcohol, tobacco, prescription) and stress level.

How was your diet as an infant? As a child? A developing brain is highly dependent on proper nutrition on an ongoing basis to supply the necessary building blocks during many brain growth spurts.

Did you enjoy the benefits of being highly stimulated (emotionally) as a child? Supportive parental care assures growth of the hippocampus, the section of the brain most vulnerable to neuron loss as AD progresses.

Were you raised in a large family? Being raised in a large family increases the chances of AD, as parental emotional support is divided between many children, inhibiting hippocampus growth, similar to being placed in daycare.

Location: did you enjoy the benefits of the same location as a child? Moving around as a child puts much stress on the brain, as you have to adapt to new environments and friends. This creates much plasticity (reorganization of neurons and connecting synapses) at a most vulnerable time.

Divorce is devastating to a child's brain! Great neuron networks are created through a family united, with divorce bringing much plasticity as one is switched from one environment to another. Were you raised in a dysfunctional family? Many parents do not take the path of a legal divorce but divorce emotionally. Just as devastating to a child, if not more so, as they witness the constant battles, enduring much stress.

As a child there is a tremendous level of chemicals and growth factors solely dedicated to the development of the brain. The world around you as a child determines which neurons and connections are going to remain and which ones will be pruned away, leaving you with a basic foundation for life.

How do you measure up? Rate your childhood.

Conception to birth

Mother's diet

a. Balanced (nutritional)	3
b. High carbohydrate	-1
c. High protein	-1
d. Low-Low fat	-2
e. High fat diet (junk food)	-2
f. Artificial sweeteners	-1

Stress level

a. Supportive husband	1
b. Supportive family	1
c. Single parent	-1
d. Job	-1
e. Stressful job	-2

Drug use

a. Heavy caffeine use (soda, coffee, chocolate, etc.)	-1
b. Alcohol consumption	-1
c. Heavy use of alcohol	-2
d. Illegal drug use	-1 through -3

Total

Birth till age 3 years

Birth

a. Normal	1
b. Planed caesarian	1
c. Traumatic birth	-1
d. Premature	-2

Diet

a. Naturally breastfed	2
b. Bottled breast milk	1
c. Nutritional diet	1

d. Poor diet   -1

Nurturing

a. Full time nurturing mom	2
b. Two supportive parents	1
c. Supportive extended family	1
d. Daycare	-1
e. Poor daycare	-2
f. Lack of nurturing (feelings of loneliness)	-2
g. Stressful family environment	-2

Sleep

a. 12 hours per day	1
b. 8 hours or less	-1

Total

Childhood in general

Diet

a. Balanced diet (nutritional)	2
b. Sporadic diet	-1
c. Poor diet	-2
d. Artificial sweeteners	-1
e. High in fat (junk food)	-1

Nurturing

a. Two supportive parents	2
b. Single parent home (non-nurturing)	-1
c. Supportive extended Family	1
d. Non related mentor	1
e. Abusive	-1
f. Sexually abusive	-2

Family

a. Siblings 1-3	1
b. Sibling 4-6	-1
c. More then 6	-2
d. Parental divorce	-1
e. Lack of contact after divorce	-1
f. Happily remarried (supportive stepparent)	1

Health

a. Generally healthy	1
b. Poor health	-1
c. Allergies	-1
d. Obesity	-1
e. Diabetic	-3
f. Head injury	-3

Sleep

a. 8-10 hours per day	1
b. Less then 7 hours	-1

Drug use

a. Heavy caffeine use (soda, coffee, chocolate, etc.)   -1

b. Alcohol consumption   -1

c. Heavy use of alcohol   -2

d. Illegal drug use   -1 through -5

e. Artificial sweeteners   -1

Location

a. Same childhood location   2

b. Change of location   -1

c. Many changes of location   -2

d. Relocate rural to urban (mid-childhood)   -2

e. Toxic location   -2

General

a. Optimistic   1

b. Pessimistic   -1

c. Depressed   -1

d. Manic depressive   -2

e. Physically active (sports)   2

f. Socially active   1

Total

Age 20-50 years

For 20 years others have been controlling the forces that determine your vulnerability to AD. As an adult now, you control your diet, relationships with others, and choice of job. Choose them wisely.

If you enjoyed the benefit of a healthy diet when you were young, continue it. If not, you now control your diet. Take control; help lessen your chances of going down the AD path.

Most laugh at the fact that a male will choose a spouse similar to his mother and a female similar to her dad. But it is something that is most healthy in re-enforcing childhood foundations. Choose your mate wisely and enjoy the benefits of a healthy marriage. Continue the benefits of an ongoing family relationship. Even a once dysfunctional family can mend its difficulties and move on in a positive way.

Over the next 30 years your job will consume one-third of your time, therefore having much control over your vulnerability to AD. Turning your childhood goals into reality is most beneficial. Taking the path others have chosen for you is not. Take control over your job; don't let it take control over you. Enjoy the benefit of a 24-hour day: 8 hours work, 8 hours pleasure, and 8 hours sleep. Use the 48-hour weekend to help you compensate when times get tough. Most of us only get one chance at choosing an occupation. Choose it wisely and enjoy. Don't let it become a driving force in increasing your vulnerability to AD.

Diet

a. Balanced (nutritional)	2
b. Sporadically balanced	1
c. Poor diet	-1
d. High carbohydrate	-1
e. High protein	-1
f. Low, low fat diet	-2
g. High in fat (junk food)	-1
h. Artificial sweeteners	-1

Relationships

a. Ongoing supportive parents	1
b. Close immediate family ties	3
c. Continuation of childhood friendships	2
d. Socially active (not out of depression)	2
e. Happily married through life	2
f. Ongoing positive relationship with children	2
g. Single through life (many partners)	-1
h. No relationship with others	-1
i. Divorce	-2
j. Happily remarried	1
k. No relation with children after divorce	-2
l. Ongoing positive sexual relations	2

Job

a. Continuation of childhood goal	3
b. Enjoy job	2
c. Hate job	-1
d. Continuous job stress (that's not dealt with)	-1
e. Traumatic change of occupation	-2
f. Continuous exposure to toxin	-2 through -10
g. Physical job	1

Health

a. Generally healthy	2
b. Poor health	-1

c. Allergies	-1
d. Obesity	-1
e. Diabetic	-3
f. Head injury	-3
g. Heart or artery disease	-3

Sleep

a. 8-10 hours per day	1
b. Less then 7 hours	-1

Drug use

a. Heavy caffeine use (soda, coffee, chocolate, etc.)	-1
b. Moderate alcohol consumption (2 glasses wine, 2 beers, 1 liquor)	2
c. Heavy use of alcohol	-2
d. Illegal drug use	-1 through -3
e. Moderate consumption caffeine	1
f. Continuous estrogen replacement therapy	4
g. Continuous use of anti-inflammatory drugs (non-steroid)	3

Location

a. Same as childhood	2
b. Change of location	-1
c. Many changes of location	-2
d. Relocate rural to urban	-2
e. Toxic location	-2

General

a. Optimistic	2
b. Pessimistic	-2
c. Depressed	-1
d. Manic depressive	-3
e. Physically active	2
f. Continuation of childhood sports	3
g. Continuation of childhood hobbies	2
h. Socially active	2

Total

Age 50 till death

If others and yourself have made wise choices for the first 50 years of life, one should enjoy the next 50 years free of AD. If not so wise, it's never too late to turn it around. Harness the wisdom you have gained over the years and take control, before AD takes control of you. Latch on to a balanced nutritional diet. Start re-enforcing your relationship with others (most important, family) and start weaning yourself from your job. Don't look at it as if the glass is now half empty but half full—full of many more years of happiness if you would just take control.

Diet

a. Balanced (nutritional)	3
b. Sporadically balanced	1
c. Poor diet	-1
d. High carbohydrate	-2
e. High protein	-2
f. Low, low fat diet	-3

g. High in fat (junk food)   -1
h. Cholesterol controlling diet   2
i. Artificial sweeteners   -1
j. Heavy use of artificial sweeteners   -2
k. Sporadic food consumption   -1

Relationships

a. Ongoing supportive parents   1
b. Close immediate family ties   3
c. Continuation of childhood friendships   2
d. Socially active (not out of depression)   2
e. Happily married through life   2
f. Ongoing positive relationship with children   2
g. Single through life (many partners)   -1
h. No relationship with others   -1
i. Divorce   -2
j. Happily remarried   1
k. No relation with children after divorce   -2
l. Ongoing positive sexual relations   2

Job

a. Continuation of childhood goal   3
b. Enjoy job   2
c. Hate job   -1
d. Continuous job stress (that's not dealt with)   -1
e. Traumatic change of occupation   -2
f. Continuous exposure to toxin   -2 through 10

g. Physical job   1

Retirement

a. Remained physically active   2
b. Remained cognitively active   2
c. Socially active (not out of depression) 2
d. Continuation of job skills (volunteer, part-time)   3
e. Complete change of stimulate (life) * (loss, retirement, change of location)   -1 through –20

Health

a. Generally healthy   2
b. Poor health   -1
c. Allergies   -1
d. Obesity   -1
e. Diabetic   -3
f. Head injury   -3
g. Heart or artery disease   -3

Sleep

a. 7-8 hours per day   1
b. Less then 6 hours   -1

Drug use

a. Heavy caffeine use (soda, coffee, chocolate, etc.)   -1
b. Moderate alcohol consumption (2   2

glasses wine, 2 beers, 1 liquor)

c. Heavy use of alcohol	-3
d. Illegal drug use	-3
e. Moderate consumption caffeine	1
f. Estrogen replacement therapy	4
g. Continuous use of anti-inflammatory drugs (non-steroid)	3

Location

a. Same as childhood	2
b. Return to similar childhood location	2
c. Change of location (negative)	-1
d. Many changes of location	-2
e. Toxic location	-2

General

a. Optimistic	2
b. Pessimistic	-2
c. Depressed	-1
d. Manic depressive	-3
e. Physically active	2
f. Continuation of childhood sports	3
g. Continuation of childhood hobbies	2
h. Socially active	1

Total

* An abrupt change of stimulus can be devastating on the mind. You are highly dependent on the environmental stimulants you have created around you in exciting the brain every day, assuring

its survival. Abrupt changes like spousal loss, retirement and change of location can quickly take you down the path of AD. Seek out other sources of past environmental stimulants to keep your brain excited, find new forms of environmental stimulants and move on.

Genetics

Half of your vulnerability to Alzheimer's is laced within your ApoE 2-3 or 4 gene. You inherit one from each parent. Having inherited two ApoE2 genes will much lessen your chance of AD. While two ApoE4 genes will very much increase your vulnerability. Or you could be anywhere in between. With the high cost of gene testing today, you can probably only guess your gene type. Here are some helpful hints:

1. Observe other family members. Do both of your parents' families seem to enjoy a long life free of AD, and good health in general? If so, you probably inherited two ApoE2 genes. If you observe AD on both sides of the family tree you probably inherited two ApoE4 genes.

2. After years of research, I would have to hypothesize your ongoing memory is very much related to gene type: ApoE2 creating a strong memory, ApoE4 very weak. How do you compare?

3. Another role carried out by ApoE is the assisting of the transportation within the body of cholesterol. Are you one of the lucky ones, who can pretty much eat anything you like and still not gain weight? You probably inherited two ApoE2 genes. Or are you the type of individual where that bag of potato chips goes straight to your hips (ApoE4)?

Genetics

a. ApoE2-ApoE2   50
b. ApoE2-ApoE3   45

c. ApoE2-ApoE4	35
d. ApoE3-ApoE3	40
e. ApoE3-ApoE4	30
f. ApoE4-ApoE4	25

Total

Add up your score. If you surpassed 100 you should enjoy a life free of AD. On average, scores under 100 will come pretty close to age of onset. With so many factors involved, truly predicting one's age of onset is most difficult. This test has been devised from years of observing others, with its values only being estimated. Only by scientific study can we turn estimates into accurate values.

NOTE: If you are under age 50, or barely into your 50s or 60s, to avoid confusion in taking this Alzheimer's Self-Test, base your answers on a personal prediction of your future diet and environmental stimulants. Very often your past habits will follow you throughout life. If you don't like the test results, evaluate your answers and determine what changes you need to make in your life to prevent Alzheimer's. It is never too late to make changes for the better.

"Children are the living messages we send to a time we will not see."

John W. Whitehead

Chapter 3: Before and after the cradle

The best place and time to begin disease-proofing your children is when they are fetuses in the womb. It's just a matter of common sense. What the mother ingests does affect the fetus, either positively or negatively. The fetus can be given a head start on life or handicapped for life.

What it boils down to is whether the parent is willing to take full responsibility to do everything possible to assure optimum pre-natal as well as post-natal health. To some, upon realizing that they are pregnant, this might mean giving up cigarettes and going slow on caffeine. To others it might mean avoiding alcohol or drugs or both. And to all it means staying away from radiation, usually in the form of x-rays.

Getting on and staying on a good, well-balanced diet throughout the pregnancy is definitely in the best interest of the fetus.

Chances are strong that the mother's overall health will also benefit from whatever positive ingesting habits are formed.

And stay away from aspartame!

Everybody's health would benefit by eliminating sweeteners; however, the best possible of all times to trash aspartame-laced products is during pregnancy.   If you didn't already, you now know that **aspartame is poison**. It is the kind of product that the skull and crossbones symbol was made for. Every item that has aspartame in it should display the skull and crossbones.

Would you knowingly feed poison to yourself, spouse, child, or that future adult in your womb?

Don't be one of those people who let selfishness override common sense. Let go of any habit that might interfere with your health or anyone's health in your family. Start by kicking the aspartame habit.

In most homes children use sugarless products just as much as adults. Some-times a parent will feed aspartame products to a child in the belief that by eliminating the sugar that the child will become less hyperactive. Perhaps it is done with the goal of making a child less obese. Many times the products are there because the parent is on a weight-loss diet.

Start checking the contents of the products that you buy. If the word aspartame or sweetener is included, look for a substitute product. Even some baby formulas have aspartame. That, in my opinion, is a high crime.

Common products that are laced with this poison include instant breakfasts, breath mints, cereals, sugar-free chewing gum, cocoa mixes, coffee beverages, frozen desserts, gelatin desserts, juice beverages, laxatives, multivitamins, milk drinks, pharmaceuticals and supplements, shake drinks, tabletop sweeteners, tea beverages, instant teas and coffees, topping mixes, wine coolers, and even yogurt.

Diet drinks are major conduits of aspartame.

Again, get in the habit of reading product contents.

If the only good that came out of people reading this book was that they stopped poisoning themselves and their family with aspartame, then writing this book would be worthwhile. You have the knowledge. What are you going to do with it?

First three years are so important

When a child is born there are 100 billion neurons and trillions of connections waiting to be nurtured. If you nurture your child properly during the first three years after birth, about one-half of those neurons and connections will be pruned during natural processes.

Back in the days when mom stayed home and took care of her own children nurturing was not a problem. Most of those kids turned out just fine.

But times and routines have changed. Today, mom takes a leave from work, gives birth, then perhaps stays home to love and nurture her baby for maybe six weeks. Then it's back to work as usual and little baby is dumped into a five-to-one ratio daycare center staffed by minimum wage caregivers whose main goal in life is just to survive from paycheck to paycheck.

Baby has gone from a one-to-one nurturing ratio to a five-to-one setting in which truly nurturing caregivers are rare.

BAM!

Just like that the baby, because of the plunge in nurturing quality, might face the loss of an additional twenty-five percent of the neurons and connections. That means the potential of having only one-fourth of the neurons and connections left to last for a lifetime. That's not much protection against the onset of diseases later in life.

What harm can the daycare routine really do?

I'm glad that you asked. Let's go back to those first six weeks that baby has mom's full attention and devotion. All those large neuro networks are forming nicely and they are getting the environmental stimuli needed to assure their continued growth.

Then an abrupt change occurs. Those neuro networks no longer are getting the encouragement of consistent stimuli. Baby starts to receive stimulus from other people, often several others during the course of one day.

What neuroscientists call plasticity takes place creating new circuits and other networks based on the stimuli from the caregivers. Baby, although so very young, begins to experience confusion. It's a strange new environment and all the baby's senses kick in. The scents and sights of mother whom the baby was introduced to at birth are no longer a constant.

If baby were able to speak, we might hear questions like, "Who is my mother? Is it this person who is taking care of me today? Or is it the person who wakes me up, drops me off at this place, then picks me up late in the day, gives me a bath, and puts me to bed?"

Then comes the weekend. Suddenly the baby is getting some good old-fashioned nurturing and lots of personal attention. Neuron reinforcement begins all over only to be interrupted again on Monday when baby is thrust back into the five-to-one ratio routine.

In all but the rare cases where the caregiver really is good at nurturing, the baby will have more neurons and networks pruned than is desirable. Factor in the situations where diet is poor and there is family discord and lots of stress, and then potential problems are compounded.

Nurturing is a BIGGIE

The consistent loving care that a child is given during those first three foundational years is the most important factor of all. Nothing can match the positive effectiveness of that one-to-one parent-child match-up.

Many times I have had parents tell me, "But my child has everything." Yes. The child has everything that money can buy. The purchase of shoes every week might fulfill the parents' needs. But the child's needs are better met if you are there to put them on, be there to tie them during the day, and be there to take them off at night.

All the things you buy for the very young child do not have any value unless you are there to share them with your child. You cannot buy love. But you can show it. Even if you're a parent caught up in the daycare trap, you can figure out how to come up with the time necessary to give the proper nurturing that your child deserves.

Take a look at the monkeys

Monkeys in the wild nurture their young for as long as six years never letting the offspring out of their sight. Yet we say that we as humans are more intelligent than the monkey. Maybe we are when it comes to inventing things. But are we really when it comes to nurturing our young?

Monkeys don't develop AD (except with one exception which we'll get to in a moment). Doesn't that make you wonder why?

They live a consistent life with very little change. They nurture their young and maintain family units for life, always caring for the young and the other members of their particular family unit. Aunts, uncles, nieces, brothers, sisters, nephews, mate, close friends, they all stick together through whatever comes their way, good times and bad.

They suffer little disease.

Now let's discuss that exception that I mentioned. Monkeys, too, can develop AD if they are abandoned and not stimulated or defeated by a dominant male. The testosterone level in the defeated male drops as much as eighty percent within one day after the defeat. The victim becomes very docile, depressed and vulnerable to stress out of fear of another defeat.

Monkeys need the consistent nurturing provided by their family units.

Do you see a lesson in there somewhere? I hope so.

A plan to fight drugs and other stimulants

This is as good a place as any to have this discussion. So here it is.

As a parent or guardian, you are responsible for your child's pleasurable experiences in life. Don't let them replace those pleasures with drugs, alcohol, tobacco, or other artificial stimulants.

Children need attention and pleasurable experiences to deter them from choosing the path of abusive substances. You have control of your own pleasurable experiences but your child does not. Remember that you are in charge. You really can use preventative methods to help keep your children substance-free. I will share with you a plan that has worked well for most people who have tried and stuck with it.

Your life expectancy is about seventy-five years, and all that you need to make is an investment of about three percent of your life to properly stimulate your child. That works out to about three hours a day for the first eighteen years of your child's life.

But guess what? That leaves ninety-seven percent of your life to do with as you choose. What a deal! Just three hours a day to help assure that your child enjoys a drug-free childhood.

The plan requires one hour in the morning and two hours in the afternoon and evening. Follow this plan and I guarantee you that years from now both you and your child will have fond memories of those "together times."

Consistently give your child positive attention and pleasurable experiences and it will pay rich dividends during the rest of both your lives. One of the by-products for some families is the elimination of depression. Interesting.

OK. Here's the plan. Well, actually it's a list of simple suggestions of ways to pleasure your child.

WEEK DAYS

Morning: One hour

Wake up your child with a kiss on the forehead.

Help your child pick out clothes for the day.

Help your child pick up his or her room. (If you do this every day it will take less than ten minutes and will stop future arguments.)

Take time out for yourself while your child gets ready for school. Prepare yourself for work or enjoy something that you like to do.

Enjoy a healthy breakfast with your child. Rotate your meals through the week: fruits, cereals, eggs, bacon, and pancakes. A child needs all food groups to assure optimum health and so do you. Enjoy preparing and cleaning up together. One morning a week let your child fix breakfast for you, something simple; you can clean up while your child watches a favorite morning show. Surprise your child! Use a red marker and draw a big heart on your child's mirror instructing to meet you at the front door at 7:30 a.m. (or whatever time will work in your case). Go out for breakfast at the child's favorite place even if it is McDonald's.

Brush your child's hair or help choose the right makeup.

Give your child a kiss and hug good-bye and send him or her off to school.

If you pack lunch, insert a little hello note or I love you message.

Follow these eight steps in a consistent manner and it will be all that your child needs to start the day on a positive note. A bonus is that your child's room will stay clean and picked up and so will the kitchen. That means you will have less to worry about or argue about later.

Afternoon or Evening: Two hours

With today's busy lifestyle and often the need for two family incomes, many children feel alone and lack attention, especially after school. Schedule adult supervision for your child or make arrangements for participation in an after-school program with many pleasurable activities.

Encourage young adults in your community to baby-sit, especially if it is someone that your child and his or her peers look up to. This will provide jobs for local youth and keep them out of trouble and well stimulated in a positive way.

Have the young adult help your child with homework, as he or she will usually be more familiar with today's method of teaching modern math and computers.

Schedule pleasurable activities after completion of homework.

Let the babysitter go somewhere special with your child once a week as a reward for good behavior.

When you return home from work, your child's room should be clean and picked up from that morning and the homework should be done. Again, this will eliminate the most common argument amongst parent and child, leaving only pleasure and time to enjoy and relax yourself, and time you can share with your child.

Have dinner with your family and children at least twice a week. Help the children prepare a special dinner they have chosen for themselves and enjoy with them.

Check over your child's homework making sure that it has been completed. Don't correct it – you will be criticizing your child. That is the teacher's job, not yours. If corrections are needed, instruct the teacher that your child needs help in that area. If the teacher doesn't respond or have time to respond due to large classroom size, instruct the babysitter to help, or hire a tutor who will make the child feel special, as he or she will be receiving more attention.

Discuss with your child how the day went and what pleasurable things happened during the day.

Relax and enjoy the rest of the evening yourself. Just don't forget to tuck your child into bed and give a kiss and hug goodnight. This will help them close the day on the same positive note you started them on.

WEEKENDS

Three hours per day

By working with your child during the week, you have taught responsibility and good health. Your child can prepare and clean up after his or her own breakfast while you sleep in. Consistent patterns during the week will bring consistent results on the weekend.

Put your weekend schedule on the refrigerator, leaving a space so that your child can also put up a schedule. Leave one hour open in your schedule for your child to choose a joint activity such as lunch or dinner, or maybe just some time to throw a ball back and forth.

Reward the child with what was chosen on the schedule if he or she has completed all the tasks during the week.

Children need to feel important and needed. Let them write their own grocery list, for when they fix your breakfast during the week, and what they would like for lunch and one dinner during the week especially for them. Take them shopping with you and let them get the items on their list. It will keep them occupied and out of trouble in the supermarket. Also, it will teach them responsibility and finance. Give older children a budget to follow.

For children who participate in sports, don't just drop them off, but watch them or better yet volunteer your time. You are the one most important in your children's lives, and you are the one they want to impress the most.

ENJOY!

Follow these helpful hints and you can enjoy a most pleasurable experience with your child or children. Chances are very good that you will not have to worry about drugs, alcohol, or smoking. Consistency is the key. If you miss a day or so don't worry or try and make up for it, just continue from where you left off. Be as consistent as your lifestyle will allow.

But I must warn you that this plan comes with a disclaimer. There is one side effect: your children will receive enough love and attention during the day that they will no longer have to act out or misbehave to get attention.

Chapter Three: Key points to remember

The best of all possible times to trash aspartame-laced products is during pregnancy.

The first three years are tremendously important in a child's development.

Children that receive consistent, positive nurturing while growing up, have stronger immune systems to defend against disease.

The three-hour-a-day plan generates results and memories that will last a lifetime.

"Your family is what you've got…It's your limits and your possibilities. Sometimes you'll get so far away from it you'll think you're outside its influence forever, then before you figure out what's happening, it will be right beside you, pulling the strings. Some people get crushed by their families. Others are saved by them."

Peter Collier

Chapter 4: Maximize family ties

A classic study done during the mid-1970s showed the importance of family as a factor in disease prevention.

Leonard Syme, Ph.D., compared 17,000 Japanese men who lived in California and Japan. He focused on cholesterol levels and rates of heart disease. One of his assumptions going into the study was that high cholesterol levels served as a good marker for the probability of heart disease.

But what he found caught him by surprise. Even though their counterparts living in Japan had similar cholesterol levels, the Japanese men living in California had five times the rate of heart disease. And when Dr. Syme went a step further and compared the study groups in regard to blood pressure, cigarette smoking, and other heart disease indicators, the Japanese men living in California still had two to five times the rate of heart disease as did the men in Japan.

What in the world was going on?

Dr. Syme went to Japan to find out. He quickly had the answer. "Japanese society is organized around social networks much tighter than what we have in the U.S. Japanese people still have very close ties to their families, neighborhoods, and jobs. To Americans, that looks claustrophobic, like an invasion of privacy.

But to the Japanese, our mobile, individualistic lifestyle looks terribly lonely, rootless, and isolated."

The surprising results of that study led Dr. Syme to conclude that maintaining close social ties had a "protective" effect in regard to disease prevention.

The opposite effect has many times been substantiated in cases of isolation, that is, where there is an absence of social ties (family). Studies have shown that social isolation releases a flood of stress hormones into the blood that trigger many psychological and physiological changes, including impaired immune function and feelings of depression and anxiety.

Support groups reduce isolation

In today's fast-paced society it is common for families to be strewn about the country. It would practically take an Act of Congress or God (death of a family member) to get everybody back together and then it's usually just long enough to say hi and good-bye. Then it's right back to the rut of multiple jobs and daycare centers, with stress being piled upon stress.

One means that is being touted more and more to combat isolation is the concept of support groups. Which is probably a good thing if you or some member of your family is serving as a caregiver for someone with Alzheimer's. The support group serves as an emotional outlet, a means of seeing for your self that you are not alone in the task you are doing.

Now I've got to jump on my soapbox. Because, you see, if people knew about Dr. Syme's study soon after the results were in, and those people took to heart the message of the study – that families are important – then there would be fewer cases of AD today. Which would mean there would be less need for support groups, and fewer people would have to be caregivers.

Consider the case of Ronald Reagan

Have you ever wondered why the former President became a victim of AD? I believe that if he were able to participate in the questionnaire in the last chapter of this book a pattern would develop showing traumatic events that triggered the isolation and eventual destruction of massive neuron networks in his brain.

Keep in mind what we've discussed about the benefits of close family ties.

Now what AD markers might stick out in Mr. Reagan's personal history?

His family at one point broke up for about a year.
Went through a very emotionally draining divorce.
Didn't talk much with one son for two decades.
With re-marriage, made new associations while giving up others.
Carried hurts regarding relationship with a daughter.
Had a career change that brought with it much stress.

Any one or all of these might have been among the factors that led Mr. Reagan on the path toward AD. The seeds of AD could have been planted during his childhood. He was raised by an alcoholic father. And to cope, at a very young age he learned how to suppress memory. That suppression of memory continued throughout his life, even into his presidency: living in denial over Iran's arms for hostages and the contra scandal that almost took him down. His would be a most interesting personal history to study.

While we're in the neighborhood

One factor I'd like to know about Mr. Reagan's past is his sleep pattern history. The reason for sleep is to restore energy and bring the body back into balance. Lack of sleep alters hormones and metabolism. When the lack of sleep is chronic, odds for serious problems down the road increase greatly.

Before I tell you about a fascinating study, yes, I do believe that chronic sleep disorder is a possible marker for the later onset of AD. It can really play havoc with your immune system.

Results of the study by researchers from the University of Chicago Medical Center were published in the October 23, 1999 issue of *The Lancet.*

Eleven healthy young men were allowed varying hours of sleep over sixteen days. All were given identical diets. They slept 11 p.m. to 7 a.m. – eight hours – on the first three nights. Over the following six nights they were put on a sleep deprivation schedule of four hours from 1 a.m. to 5 a.m. Then for seven days they stayed in bed for twelve hours from 9 p.m. until 9 a.m.

Tests were administered to all participants at specific times during the sixteen days. Major alternations of glucose metabolism occurred during sleep deprivation. Subjects took forty percent longer than normal to regulate their blood sugar levels after eating a high carbohydrate meal. Their ability to secrete and respond to insulin decreased by about thirty percent. That usually is an early marker of diabetes.

Sleep deprivation also changed production and action of other hormones, including secretion of thyroid stimulating hormone, and increasing levels of cortisol. Elevated cortisol levels are a factor in AD progression.

All of the abnormalities returned to baseline (normal) and beyond during the recovery period when subjects stayed in bed twelve hours. This means that more than eight hours of daily rest might be needed for young adults to function at optimum levels.

The nine hours sleep that Americans averaged in 1910 had eroded to seven-and-one-half hours by 1975. With today's millions of shift workers getting only about five hours sleep, that 1975 average has trended even lower.

And the lower that average goes, the higher grows the percentage of people getting various diseases, including AD.

Here's a little getting-to-sleep trick

It's easier to enjoy and foster family togetherness when each family member is well rested at the start of a new day.

One trick I've learned is how to regulate melatonin that is produced in the brain and triggers sleep. A few hours before going to sleep I start turning down the lights. Then, about an hour before hitting the sack, I turn off all lights except for the low light coming from the computer or TV.

This progression of less and less light simulates nature, and when I finally do go to bed my body has the correct level of melatonin. I'm headed for deep, refreshing sleep in about five minutes and do not toss and turn during the night.

A light on a rheostat works great.

Keep family ties going for life

What brings the most joy to millionaires?

According to Thomas Stanley, who surveyed 733 millionaires while writing his book, *The Millionaire Mind*, one of their biggest kicks comes from watching their children or grandchildren playing sports.

Most of these millionaires have never been divorced and, on average, have been married for 28 years to the same spouse. Above all, they have a love for life.

As millionaires have a choice of stimulants, being so involved with family, children, and grandchildren must be very stimulating to the mind. They have found the key to keeping their minds stimulated, and exciting massive amounts of neurons to keep their minds strong.

Watching children or grandchildren perform in sports, especially when the child's team wins, raises testosterone levels. In males, testosterone produces estrogen, and estrogen is a factor in helping prevent AD.

The feeling a father or grandfather gets, for example, watching the child score a goal is the next best thing to orgasm in stimulating positive effects for the whole body.

Married people less likely to develop AD

Findings of a study done at Bordeaux University in France indicate that never-married individuals have "a twofold increase for the risk of dementia and almost a threefold increase for the risk of Alzheimer's disease."

A married person receives constant stimulation of the hippocampus, which is the area of the brain that suffers most from AD. In a happy marriage built on love and not on convenience, as so many marriages are built on today, one receives much emotional support whether it is good (pleasure) or bad (pain) to prevent degeneration and apopotosis from today's rat race pace.

Happily married couples pass those traits down to their children, helping to create a strong family unit.

The power of love

You've probably heard about someone who was diagnosed with a disease from which the medical people said there was little or no chance for recovery. Then something miraculous happened and the patient recovered.

In many cases the "miracle" was due to the power of love.

Love has the power to organize one's hormones and chemicals in performing unbelievable feats of strength to save a loved one, a child for example.

Love is the most powerful force in human nature. I believe it is a force that should receive priority over all other research. But at this point I'd be surprised if it consisted of even a tenth of a percent of research, if that much.

The love factor has been a part of my research from the beginning. I only wish that I had the proper research facility available to me to conduct the right research to discover what hormonal and chemical changes take place in the body as one switches from one stimulant to another.

Conducting an appropriate study would be quite simple. It would involve testing and taking hormonal and chemical results just before divorce, and then repeating the tests right after and during the subjects' first year of marriage.

Only by doing this will confirmation be made as to what hormonal and chemical changes are actually taking place. Then we would be much better equipped to show people how to build and rebuild their immune systems. More people would have immune systems so powerful that they could overcome unbelievable odds in fighting disease.

You can take a step in that direction right now by maximizing your positive family ties.

Chapter Four: Key points to remember

People with strong, healthy family ties are less likely to end up with disease.

Married people are less likely to develop AD than unmarried people.

Long periods of sleep deprivation can set you up for disease. Eight hours' sleep, consistently, will help build your immune system.

Love is the most powerful force in human nature.

"Love does not consist in gazing at each other but in looking together in the same direction."

Antoine De Saint Exupery

"Age doesn't protect you from love.   But love, to some degree, protects you from age."

Jeanne Moreau

Chapter 5: Reinforce your mate

Positive nurturing, as pointed out two chapters ago, actually begins with the fetus in the womb. It continues through childhood on into adulthood. And right into marriage, especially the early years of marriage, when it is very important for you to reinforce your mate.

It's just common sense.

Unfortunately, as we earlier discussed, common sense has become the exception rather than the rule. Most people know what they should be doing, then go out and do the opposite. It's as if they've adopted the slogan, "Live it up today and let tomorrow take care of itself."

The problem is that when you live your life that way, you are greatly increasing the odds that when tomorrow comes you will be dependent upon a caregiver. And if you are emerged at that time in a full-blown case of Alzheimer's, you won't remember the things you did when you were living it up. You won't remember the yesterday of twenty-four hours' previous. Or even what you did a few minutes before.

Divorce and separation create stress

When mates do not positively reinforce each other consistently, there is a gradual questioning by one or both mates as to the partner's quality of devotion. The one doing the questioning usually puts out less and less effort at reinforcing the mate. When the other mate senses this, there are hurt feelings that escalate into counter questioning which leads to arguments.

Separation often follows, then divorce. An increasing number of marriage partners skip the separation phase and take the divorce pill hoping for a quick cure.

The resulting stress can create high levels of cortisol, usually at higher levels if the marriage has lasted longer rather than shorter. The neuro networks that were created no longer receive stimulation, and they start to degenerate. Especially when it is a long-term stressful relationship that has been terminated, much degeneration and apopotosis will occur.

But those individuals who are fortunate to remarry into a partnership where positive reinforcement is a goal of both mates, and there are more pleasurable stimuli, will lower their risk of becoming AD victims. This is because they are lowering their cortisol levels and increasing the size of the hippocampus through neurogenesis (the growth of new cells). They are strengthening their immune systems so beta amyloid can be dissolved before formation of the deadly tangles and plaques that we discussed in Chapter One reaches an unstoppable stage.

Someone to talk to and touch

The security in knowing that you can talk freely with your mate and have pleasurable physical contact with that person is a bonus that leads to the lowering of cortisol levels. This in turn further boosts your immune system.

The power of love that we talked about in the previous chapter is so important in developing and maintaining positive chemical supplies in your brain and throughout your body.

Human touch is so essential between mates. A kiss at every meeting or departure helps to maintain consistent hormone levels throughout the day. Back rubs and hugs are great reinforcement. Go ahead and hug your wife, squeeze those hormones out of the cells and into the bloodstream, where they can perform their jobs in maintaining bodily functions.

If one hugs an autistic child during a temper tantrum that child will calm down; very similar to the holding technique used on children with attachment disorders, while trying to get them to reattach and bond. Take a good look at today's society. You will see just as many attachment disorders among adults as there are among children; however, the adults are more adept at covering up the problem and hiding from a solution.

Many adults are afraid of attachment. They're in constant fear of another loss, which brings much pain into their lives. And so many of them have become afraid of the opposite sex. They reason that if they don't become attached to anybody they will not suffer another loss. And when such a process continues for years – sometimes for most of one's life – an erosion of neuron networks gradually takes place and finally that person is a prime candidate for disease.

How confused an individual becomes if not nurtured correctly as a child; and if one is nurtured correctly as a child, how confused that person becomes when that nurturing doesn't continue after marriage.

Such lack of nurturing leads far too many people into the arms of others whose lust at first takes on the appearance of caring. All kinds of feelings set in, among them stress caused by the fear of getting caught while having an affair.

Mates need to learn what each other's touch levels and needs are, and then adapt to them. This will lead to a harmony that can last a lifetime. Thoughts of divorce, separation, and affairs will be replaced by unconditional love, companionship, and trust.

Loss of a spouse can be an AD trigger

Many individuals become solely dependent on their spouses for emotional stimuli. Upon the death of a mate, especially if it has been a long marriage, the survivor is often reluctant to remarry. The result is that stimulation of the massive neuron network built up during the marriage ceases. In such cases AD symptoms often show up quickly.

Those people who were less dependent on stimuli from their spouses, and who enjoyed other relationships with their children or close friends, are less likely to develop AD. This is because they have other neuron networks that they can depend on to create hormonal balance. They are able to maintain proper bodily function which includes maintaining one's immune system so that it remains capable of dissolving beta amyloid even as the networks that were developed from stimuli from the deceased spouse start to degenerate.

People that never marry, rarely develop large neuron networks within the hippocampus; although they can develop many small networks through many different relationships. This leads to many changes in stimuli, causing the hippocampus to be constantly rebuilding. At the same time, degeneration and apopotosis take place, depleting the supply of chemicals necessary to rebuild and eliminate the beta amyloid. The brain can go into battle against itself and disrupt hormonal balance.

Hey, guys, listen up!

I'm going into what I call my rambling mode; however, let the words soak in and you just might find some ideas to help strengthen the romance in your marriage and build togetherness in your family.

The medical folks will have you believe that reducing stress will cure many problems. Well, hear this. Reducing stress is not the solution. Pleasure is, something that is so easy to apply and reintroduce back into your lives.

Everyone complains that they don't have the time or money. But they find the time and money after a problem occurs.

Receiving attention is essential to stimulating positive hormones. It costs only $75 (Could be less depending on where you live.) to get a room at a local motel or hotel. And it's yours from 11 a.m. one day until 11 a.m. the next day.

It costs $150 an hour for a good psychologist. $150 that one usually comes up with or puts the burden on insurance companies. Which means higher rates for you. You are going to pay one way or another. We both know that. So listen up as I show you how to profit both financially and emotionally.

Make it a surprise

Meet your wife for lunch at the motel or hotel restaurant.

(And for the wives who need control, invite your husband. But make it a surprise, as that will increase your mate's adrenaline.)

Pre-order lunch as time is of the essence. Better yet, have lunch in the room. And then sneak in a "quickie" for that touch of excitement. Just like the old days when you were first falling in love.

The experience will probably be very associative and re-excite many positive chemical-producing hormones.

You won't want to, but go back to work

All the while keep in mind that the room is yours from 11 a.m. that day until 11 a.m. tomorrow.

After work one of you go home and get the kids (That is, if you have young kids.). That will give the other one the opportunity to stay at work a little longer and earn some overtime to help pay for the room. Or, if you're self-employed, just be more productive.

Either way it means more money and taxes vital to keep the economy going. Not to mention the money you spend at the hotel.

Have dinner with your spouse and children. Having together times as a family is very important, especially in ways that bring pleasure.

If you have a child that misbehaves use the hotel's swimming pool as positive leverage. The kid will sit there like a little angel knowing the reward for being good; also, those veggies that you spend night after night trying to cram down the child's throat will disappear.

Providing your child or children are old enough, send them to the pool and go back to your room. Only this time you don't have to make it a "quickie." Mix in a little massage. That right there will save you fifty bucks as you won't have to get it from a physical therapist each week to cut cortisol levels.

Watch the news if you must or do some work on your laptop and make some more money. While you're doing this, send your wife shopping for an hour. Many hotels and motels have little shops; and if not, some are usually close by.

Use the hotel gym to get some more necessary physical activity.

If the kids are too young to do things without your immediate supervision, schedule a babysitter who will love the pool as much as the kids do.

I almost forgot: if there's a pool available then there's usually also a hot tub nearby. Enjoy the hot tub with your spouse. Now you're getting what is known as water therapy and it is free.

Spend the night there as a family. In the morning enjoy the continental breakfast that is also free. Your wife will be refreshed, as she won't have to make beds and clean the bathroom or pick up after the kids. Someone else will do that for you.

Go back and enjoy the pool some more or get in another gym workout. Then let yourself smile, knowing that all of this cost just $75 and some well-spent change. You've also saved on gas and wear and tear on your car because you didn't have to go all over town to do these activities at different locations.

Other people will know

When you go back to work others will see pleasure radiating from your eyes and facial expressions, happiness caused by the secretion of seretonin and dopamine. And you did it without artificial stimulants or St. Johns Worts. Natural stimulation from your spouse and family did the trick. Deep down you're already thinking about ways to envelope your family in pleasure experiences.

That morning the kids will behave better in school. There will be no Ritalin needed to calm their excitement. A perceptive teacher will ask them to share with the other children the source of their happiness. Those other children in turn can pass it on to their parents as to what Johnny did last night.

Meanwhile, when others at work ask why your face is aglow, tell them what they can do for their family on just seventy-five bucks.

Who knows? Maybe we can start a positive chain reaction for once. One that is good for family health and the economy. The medical industry will suffer but they've been taking advantage of us for years only to fulfill their own greed and needs.

Keep a handle on that leverage

Your children will want to repeat the experience. Use this positive leverage you've gained to control their behavior. Reward is a very powerful mind controller. You know that from working and making money.

If you're thinking about telling me that you don't have the time and can't afford it, I don't even want to hear about it. A couple of repeat experiences and you'll save a bundle on psychological and physical therapy. And with immune systems that are getting stronger you and your family will have fewer colds and other illnesses, further saving money on doctor and medical bills.

Perhaps you need to think in investment terms

What I've given is but a limited example of the possibilities that exist to provide pleasure for yourself and your family. If you are into profit and investment opportunities, consider buying a local condo with other couples or relatives. Brothers and sisters might be best to work such a joint venture with as this provides stimulation of childhood memories.

Many condos are part of developments that include the same features that hotels and motels have, such as pools and hot tubs, even cleaning services. A good, average-size condo might run $1,000 a month or $250 a month if four people go into the deal. Now you have an investment that could bring you a nice profit later on should you sell it, but meanwhile is a good way to bring consistent doses of pleasure into your life.

If you're interested in a little extra cash flow, rent the condo out on weekends. There will also be some tax benefits to the condo ownership.

Let's take possibilities a step further

You own a small business and have several employees. The condo could serve as an excellent perk for them. Reward them for special achievement by giving them a day off to spend with their family in your condo. The kids can enjoy the pool just like they would at a hotel.

While your employees' families are getting pleasurable experiences, as a business owner you will earn dividends in the form of more work production and fewer days lost due to illness and excuses. It's a win-win situation.

Should you live in a warm climate close to the ocean or other large body of water, and you are an ambitious thinker, perhaps you might want to buy a small yacht. Just think how motivating those perks will be.

We will revisit and expand on the benefits of pleasure in one's life in Chapter Thirteen.

Chapter Five: Key points to remember

It is important that mates use positive reinforcement (nurturing) with each other.

Human touch, including massage, hugs, and kisses, builds up the immune system.

Being creative in ways that you can surprise your spouse and children with special, pleasure-filled events reaps positive dividends.

"**The family is our refuge and spring-board; nourished on it, we can advance to new horizons. In every conceivable manner, the family is link to our past, bridge to our future.**"

Alex Haley

"**The older I get the more pretty girls I remember kissing as a young man.**"

84-year-young man

Chapter 6: Keep in contact with your past

Here is a new word to add to your vocabulary:

Friendsology (noun): **a**. the process of looking for friends that one has had for many years; **b**. the renewal of association with friends from the past.

Right! One who practices **Friendsology** would be a **Friendsologist**. It makes sense to me. The concept popped into my mind while thinking about what to include in this chapter.

Like building a defensive shield

Keeping in contact with your past is a positive way of raising the odds against your becoming an AD victim in the future. Some people like to go way back in the past, as far as possible, creating family trees and learning about recent and distant ancestry. For such endeavors there are many helpful sites on the World Wide Web; for example, Genealogy@SierraHome, which offers software aids that might open up more ancestral background than you ever wanted to know.

But for this discussion, we'll mainly be talking about your personal past, things you've experienced, friends you've known.

Individuals just glow when talking about old friends. This is because neurons are getting re-excited that have been idle for years. The memories usually expand as recalling one event leads to the recalling of another, and so on, causing more neurons to get excited.

The bottom line is that it can be very beneficial to look up old friends and renew association with them, especially while you still have enough neurons left for excitation to occur.

A sad truth is that neuron networks created because of long-ago friendships are possibly the most vulnerable to apopotosis (cell death). When long periods of time elapse between contacts with those friends, the cells do not receive the stimulation needed for continued good functioning health and the danger of those cells starting to die off becomes very real.

So what are you waiting for? Take a reading break right now and get in touch with that old friend you've been meaning to contact but just haven't gotten around to it. Odds are that both of you will be glad you went to the effort.

Many ways to re-excite neurons

Here are fourteen possibilities to choose from. As you read these suggestions you will probably think of other ways that will work for you.

One: Consider a return to gardening. This is a great activity for both sufferers of Parkinson's as well as AD. It has been documented to improve the physical capabilities of PD victims and relieve motor neuron stress in those with AD. Many senior citizens were forced to garden as children during war years as a practical form of survival. Gardening now will actually help them to invigorate, possibly even save old neuron networks because of the memories that they will recall. For those who have moved from rural to urban areas, gardening reinforces memory. One potential big plus is that you can grow food in your own private garden that is non-toxic.

Two: War memorials have the power to reinforce memories, thus helping to keep neuron networks alive and well. This fact was driven home to me during a recent trip that my wife, Sandy, and I took to Washington, D.C. We visited the Vietnam Wall, Korea, and local (D.C. veterans) WWI memorials. I have never seen such happiness in such sad places. It is one of those experiences you almost have to witness to believe that what I've just said is for real. Why not see for yourself?

Three: Sports is one of the most effective triggers of memories, both good and bad, with a mixture of pleasure and pain. One way to recapture some of those old feelings about sports participation is to coach youth. It will remind you of yourself when you were young, and of all those teammates that were so important to you. There are many sports leagues out there for all ages. So if you miss that activity and there's no physical reason to hold you back, get out there and compete. For others, watching sports on TV is quite positive but not nearly as beneficial as getting off your couch and going out to see the sports activity in person. Whether it's coaching youth or being a spectator, benefits of the experience will be multiplied if your child or grandchild is involved.

Four: If you experienced abuse as a child, stop trying to suppress those memories and turn the past negative into a present positive. There are a lot of children out there who need your help. Yes, it's going to stimulate old neurons loaded with bad memories, but this activity just might be the thing that keeps a child alive. You survived and became a success in life, so share with the child that he or she, too, can become successful just like you have. By helping others you will be helping yourself.

Five: Just thinking about antiques can cause some people's brains to become awash with excited neurons. Antiques take you back into the past. Get those family heirlooms out of the basement or attic or from wherever they're stashed. Flood yourself with memories. Browse through antique stores and go to auctions where antiques are sold. Think of the possibilities, the animated conversations you are going to have with people who are also interested in antiques. Next, put that thinking into action.

Six: Cars take you to the past. Do you remember the first car you did it in? I bet that will light some neurons up. How many times have you seen an old car and the conversation quickly turns to the past? All kinds of associations will run through your mind. The car manufacturers are taking advantage, thereby stimulating more neurons, which leads to more sales. VW reintroduced the Beetle with great success. Plymouth and Dodge are selling the PT cruiser and the Prowler. Car shows are excellent surroundings in which to fire up those neurons. So is the process of doing the actual restoration of a car that you own.

Seven: If you are between occupations, consider volunteering in some capacity to help others. Or take on a part-time job in the same field as your last full-time work assignment. This will help maintain the vast networks that were created over the years. A lot of people have larger neuron networks because of their career than they do through contact with members of their own family. I believe this to be a major reason why nearly half of all men who quit working at retirement age are dead within eighteen months. They simply quit feeding massive neuron networks and did not begin any other activity that would maintain or replace those networks with new networks. Translation: keep those neurons excited.

Eight: Maintaining a history of family, friends, and past events with photos is very productive, especially if you take the time to look at the photos often. This regular unlocking of memories assures that vital neuron networks will get excited often enough to ward off cell degeneration. Reproduce photos and pass them on to family members and friends. If you're on the Internet and have a basic scanner, you can transmit photos to anyone else who's also on the Internet. With a small mini-cam or regular-size video cam you can exchange live-action scenes via the World Wide Web.

Nine: What about vacations? Have you ever revisited the same location of a past vacation that was especially stimulating? Was it a second-honeymoon-kind-of experience? Vacations can stimulate many neurons through creating conditions within the body that are ideal for neurogenesis (production of new cells) to take place. The right vacation will do wonders for rekindling the fires of passion between mates.

Ten: Music will jet you to the past with much associative stimulation. Mix in a little dancing and fine wine and you will triple the benefit. There is much documentation that physical activity and wine in moderation (one or two glasses) is good for you. Have you listened to your favorite song lately, or danced with your mate? If not, go for it.

Eleven: Many memories are highly associated with aromas: scented candles, incense, and flowers, for example. Studies have been done in which various aromas have proven to have a calming effect on those with AD. The scent of a particular perfume often is a trigger of romantic memories.

Twelve: If you have grandchildren, consider volunteering at a school or daycare center. Even if your grandkids are hundreds of miles away, you can stimulate the same neuron networks through association.

Thirteen: What better way to revisit the past than through reunions? There are family reunions, school reunions, company reunions, and other types of get-togethers that provide a good atmosphere for reinforcing neuron networks.

Fourteen: Some people have benefited from moving back to a location where they lived as children. Often those that leave an urban area to go back to a farm surrounding like that which they grew up in are happy they made the change. Some of the reasons they cite include fewer toxins, more physical activity, and friendlier neighbors. Which all adds up to less stress in one's life.

These are just suggestions. You probably have some better ones. What is important is that you keep active in ways that will keep your neuron networks strong.

Chapter Six: Key points to remember

Keeping in contact with your past can be a great way to keep those neurons excited in a most beneficial way.

It is good to recall things you've experienced, places you've been, and friends you've known.

The fourteen ways discussed to re-excite neurons are suggestions. Some might be right up your alley. If so, great. If not, think of your own hot buttons, then do something with them.

"You are never too old to set another goal or to dream a new dream."

Les Brown

"And in the end, it's not the years in your life that count. It's the life in your years."

Abraham Lincoln

Chapter 7:   Enjoy those retirement years

Use what you learn from this book to avoid becoming part of the tragic statistic mentioned in the last chapter:

About one-half of all men in the United States who work until retirement age will die on average eighteen months after they have retired.

The other half will live to their 70s, 80s, or 90s. They are the ones who did not depend primarily on their jobs for neuron stimulation. Also, they're the folks who didn't find a rocking chair and vegetate away. Their lives did not lose meaning after retirement. They simply did not fold their tents, so to speak, and give up.

Active life is very important

According to researchers involved in a recent study of post-retirement individuals with AD and those without AD, they concluded that:

Those that were less active physically and mentally were three times as likely to have AD than their more active counterparts.

The healthy study subjects were especially more active between the ages of 40 and 60. It didn't seem to matter a lot how little or how much income they had made during their careers.

In summary, the researchers' results strongly support the concept that an active life helps to prevent AD. Also, that it is never too late to get started with activities that stimulate the mind.

The "weaning" process

For purposes of our discussion, a weaning is a gradual transition between work and retirement. It can be done in any of the following three ways:

1. By changing from the full-time job just retired from to a part-time job at the same work location (which I believe is the best method).

2. Getting a part-time job or doing volunteer work in a related field at a different location.

3. Or possibly doing some consultant work which requires less commitment.

During the weaning process one has the time available to find other forms of stimulant to replace or, through association, re-stimulate and maintain neurons. Individuals who go from their jobs to chairs are the most vulnerable to either die early or develop AD, which will turn their later years into a living nightmare.

WARNING: watching TV does not lower the risk of AD.

Retirement time can be devastating on both spouses as much change takes place in the life of each mate. Routines that have been established over many years that created vast neuron networks are suddenly without benefit of consistent stimulus. If replacement activities are not already in place or not pursued, then neural regeneration can set in, setting the stage for those deadly tangles and plaques to start forming.

Add to this the new stimulus of having your spouse around all the time, and much plasticity takes place, accompanied by STRESS in capital letters. Increased stress is very common in the first few years of retirement. Often this results in the weakening of one's immune system, making that person more vulnerable for disease in general.

Some ways to get those neurons excited!

The best situation heading into retirement is to already have stimulants in place outside the work environment. But, as the researchers said, "It's never too late to get started."

Following is an outline of suggestions that can be applied to just about any occupation:

1. Military and executive

A. Consulting or part-time job in similar field
B. Involvement in other leadership positions
Politics
Local government boards
Volunteer (for example, Boy Scouts)
C. For one whose best deals were made on the golf course, continue to play.

2. Construction

A. Part-time job in area of experience
B. Open small business where you can control the number of hours you work.
C. Remodel older homes to become rental properties or for re-sale. (Dealing with tenants is easier than dealing with AD.)
D. Volunteer (for example, Habitat for housing)

E. Do all those little jobs around the house you've been putting off for years. (Stay out of your wife's hair – she needs to adapt to your being around.)

F. Hobbies.

3. Teaching

A. Substitute (Can control days you work)

B. Tutor (Your own grandchildren would be best; but if you live in different locations, use a web cam on a computer.)

C. Volunteer, for example:

Library

Adaptive grandparent program

Use your talents (story telling, puppets, music, dance, crafts, sports, safety,

occupational discussion of childhood interest, artistic)

D. Work Shops (Pass your knowledge down to others.)

E. Share a full-time job (This will assist the teacher shortage.)

F. Serve on school board or committee

4. Homemaker

A. Part-time job working with children and teens

B. Stay in contact with own children (but give them space) and grandchildren.

C. Volunteer at local schools and daycares

D. Help others with their children (part-time baby-sitting, reading writing, and arithmetic)

Yes, homemaker!

It is one of the oldest occupations in this country. And one of the highest paid jobs, not in dollars but in happiness that spreads to all the family around them. And those family members carry that happiness out into society.

In my experience I have never seen an ADD child come out of a home where mom was there nurturing that offspring properly. And rarely is the husband of such a woman depressed or stressed out at work.

Consider just two other benefits that result from the positive efforts of such moms:

There are fewer burdens on our school systems because the children of these moms are usually well behaved. And think of the money savings in terms of fewer medical and psychological problems.

It is not usually thought about, but homemakers, too, retire and do so at a very young age. There was a time when grandchildren came into the picture soon after one's children left the nest. This enabled moms to maintain neuron networks fairly easily. But that is often not the case today when increased numbers of couples delay having children due to career concerns and desires to advance educational qualifications.

So it is essential that moms find alternative methods to maintain stimulation of those vast networks created during the previous twenty to twenty-five years.

Chapter Seven: Key points to remember

An active life – before and after retirement – helps prevent Alzheimer's Disease.

The "weaning" process is important in helping people make the transition from full-time worker to active retiree.

Even homemakers go through retirement once the nest is empty.

"To learn is change. Education is a process that changes the learner."

George Leonard

Chapter 8: Plasticity: the brain's ability to adapt

Do you want the good news or the bad news first?
OK, then, here's the good news: your brain has plasticity.
Now for the bad news: your brain has plasticity.
Both statements are true.

For years the science upon which medicine is based revolved around the firm notion that the brain is hard wired. Once that wiring was completed during one's childhood, the master brain electrician's job was done.

Wrong.

Recent discoveries in the field of neuroscience have proven otherwise.

The brain is constantly rewiring itself as it adapts to the environment and individuals around it. This process is called plasticity. But mention this word to a doctor and chances are the response, after you get fixed with that queer look, will be, "No, I'm not a plastic surgeon."

The most important factor

If I had to choose one given factor as the primary cause of Alzheimer's or Parkinson's disease, I would have to say that it is the plasticity factor. One of my theories is that AD results when there is too much removal or pruning of neurons that contain painful and stressful memories. And PD is made possible by too much removal and pruning of neurons containing pleasurable memories.

Both diseases develop and progress because of negative rewiring inside the brain, which is the bad news side of plasticity.

Let's revisit life in the past

It used to be the rule that from birth to death, life was pretty consistent. Mom and dad were there to nurture you, along with all your relatives. Friends remained friends for life. And when you grew up and finally got that job you always wanted, you remained on that job permanently because if you were faithful to your employer he was faithful to you.

The same used to be true of marriage. You usually would marry your high school sweetheart and stay married until one of you died. Or, in rare cases, until one day you noticed that little Johnny bore a strong resemblance to the milkman.

Brain plasticity in those simpler times was mainly positive, which definitely was good news. Plasticity consisted of much building and strengthening of neuron networks due to consistency and repetitiveness of life.

But society has drastically changed

Society in general is not like that today. Many of us lead lives hallmarked by constant change. The majority of baby boomers have grown up with sporadic nurturing from parents, daycare employees, babysitters, step-dad, step-mom, or single parent who is doing well to know the child on a first-name basis.

What used to be the norm is now uncommon. And what used to be disdained is now considered to be a normal lifestyle. We live in a world whose values have turned upside down. So many of us jump from one relationship to another and from job to job. We also move and put our children in different schools more often.

Much negative plasticity is taking place all the time as both children and adults adapt to new environments.

Constant change creates constant plasticity.

Although change is inevitable...

We humans have been put together with brains that have the tools to facilitate change. Even while in the womb, proteasomes were available in the brain's toolbox.

The proteasomes grind up a cell's unwanted proteins and convert them to peptite fragments so that they can be removed and eventually disposed from the body as waste. An immune response is necessary to carry out this task, but in today's society the immune system is not always available to do this function. Instead, the immune system is far too often busy trying to break down too many carbohydrates or is suppressed itself due to lack of sleep or lack of proteins in one's diet.

The combined factors of too much change and the lack of an appropriate immune response can lead to the onset of AD.

Other forces are also at work

Something else besides change is causing neurons to take the path of negative plasticity in the removal of no longer needed or wanted neurons.

The enzyme presenilin plays an important role in embryonic development in helping to remove unwanted cells. Scientists believe that presenilin is somehow involved in the cutting of the amyloid precursor protein A.P.P. that appears to have a part in the forming of beta amyloid plaques and tangles. (Remember Dr. Alzheimer's discovery during the brain autopsy?)

Presenilin is made up of 467 amino acids and positioned smack dab in the middle of them are two aspartates amino acids that possibly might be very similar to the amino acids used in aspartame. When scientists removed either one of the asparates amino acids a very interesting result occurred: beta amyloid failed to appear.

Will this discovery be connected to the already overwhelming evidence that aspartame accelerates negative plasticity?

The common sense answer would be a resounding, "Yes!"

And speaking of beta amyloid

While the brain has mechanisms for connecting and preserving memories, it also has mechanisms to disconnect and remove memories.

The research of Dr. John E. Morley, chief of geriatric medicine at the St. Louis School of Medicine, has validated that the neurotransmitter beta amyloid is overproduced in the brains of Alzheimer's patients.

Dr. Morley found in animal studies that beta amyloid seems to break up memories that are no longer needed.

This is a normal, healthy process in the human brain. But when the process gets out of balance more beta amyloid will be produced than is needed. The immune system is overpowered and the beta amyloid army literally runs amok getting rid of needed memories as well as those that are no longer beneficial to keep around.

The real tragedy in all this is that most Alzheimer's cases could have been prevented through use of commonsense approaches throughout the victims' lives.

Hormones hard at work

The hormones that facilitate plasticity are at their highest performance level before puberty. After that their primary function switches gears to assist physical growth that is happening at a fast pace. Boys are often growing at such an amazing rate that you can buy new shoes for them and by the time you've reached your car in the parking lot the kid's feet have already grown one full size larger. At least it seemed that way with our sons.

As kids grow into the teen years, their mood changes sometimes assume Jeckyl and Hyde proportions. You just never know which kid is going to show up at any given time. Have you ever wondered why that is?

The answer might have been uncovered in relatively recent findings about the brain. The prefrontal cortex is still a work in progress. In fact, it is now known that this portion of the brain where emotions are rooted is not fully developed until one is about twenty years old, sometimes even a wee bit older. The brain is literally in a state of flux while the base wiring is being completed in the prefrontal cortex. While this process is going on the teen's visible, sometimes baffling behavior is but a reflection of that internal flux.

This discovery trashes the old notion that the brain is hardwired before puberty sets in.

Now for some important review

Children are born with 100 billion neurons and billions of connections and at best they are going to retain one-half of them by the age of three. The reduction of neurons is done through a very natural process called pruning.

When a greater than normal loss of neurons occurs a child's immune system is inhibited making it less able to protect the child from disease now and in later years.

In one of the studies led by Victoria Moceri, it was found that the areas of the brain that show the earliest signs of AD also take the longest time to mature during childhood and adolescence.

This finding strongly supports the need for positive plasticity. To encourage positive plasticity you don't have to read the seemingly one million books out there about stimulating your child. You just need to apply positive nurturing from birth until the child leaves your home.

The burden of responsibility

As parents, we control the probability of whether or not our children will head down the road to AD. It is not our genes; so don't use genes as an excuse. Step up to the plate and take responsibility for including prevention patterns in your life as well as the lives of your children.

If your parents did their job correctly of nurturing you during the years you lived with them, it is now your duty to maintain the good foundation given you as plasticity continues through life. Pass on that positive nurturing to your spouse and children. Increase their odds of building and maintaining strong, effective immune systems. Give them the best possible shot you can at having good health and a strong mind.

As a husband, wife, father, mother, you have great power. Use it wisely.

Chapter Eight: Key points to remember

The brain's ability to adapt to change is called plasticity, which can be a good thing or a bad thing.

Plasticity might be the primary cause of AD.

Constant change creates constant plasticity.

The combined factors of too much change and the lack of an appropriate immune response can lead to the onset of AD.

The neurotransmitter beta amyloid unconnects and removes unneeded memories; however, when hormonal imbalance sets in, beta amyloid runs amok and removes needed memories as well. As a result, beta amyloid is overproduced in the brains of Alzheimer's patients.

Most AD cases could have been prevented through use of commonsense approaches throughout the victims' lives.

"Gravitation cannot be held responsible for people falling in love."

Albert Einstein

"Put your hand on a hot stove for a minute, and it seems like an hour. Sit with a pretty girl for an hour, and it seems like a minute. THAT'S relativity."

Albert Einstein

Chapter 9: Those hard-working hormones

Did you know that sex drive and libido are important in warding off Alzheimer's Disease? I believe this to be true; however, we will discuss that in a later chapter.

The word hormone means, "to spur on" or "stir up" or "rouse."

Many people associate the word hormone with sex. And some of those people, in certain circumstances, have defensively said, "My hormones made me do it."

Two of the five hormones we are going to discuss in this chapter are universally associated with the male (testosterone) and female (estrogen) sex drives. But these hormones have other functions besides their involvement with our sexual urges. These other important functions are what we will talk about.

The other three hormones we'll be covering are cortisol, melatonin, and insulin. Yes, I said insulin, and in a few minutes you will know why.

Testosterone and estrogen

One of the many functions carried out by testosterone is development of the brain; however, through the process of aging the synthesis of testosterone by the leydig cells decreases, causing physical and mental changes. Estrogen also is important in maintaining brain function. Its depletion causes problems.

Men, as well as women, can go through menopause. It is a time when some folks pretty much give up on life. They feel they have outlived their usefulness. They withdraw from activities and associations with friends and relatives. For practical purposes they have already died. Their bodies just haven't acknowledged it yet.

Such people might as well have targets on their backs with a big D serving as the bull's eye. Because that is where the arrows of disease are headed.

Different thoughts about menopause

The age range for those men who experience menopause is considerable, from as young as thirty to as old as eighty. The typical age range for women is from forty-five to fifty-five.

Some of you readers are quite familiar with the classic symptoms including depression, irritability, reduced libido, night sweats, hot flashes, and erectile dysfunction.

My thoughts on menopause are quite different from those held by the medical community in general. I believe that menopause – especially among those men who experience the symptoms – is brought on by one's own conscious through thoughts of defeat and loss of purpose in society.

One can control the decline of both testosterone and estrogen and thereby help maintain proper brain function.

A major reason for the wide range of years in which men can experience menopause is that oftentimes at around age thirty or forty, many men get this deep-seated notion that their value to society or that their jobs as husbands are over. They've done their Tarzan thing and begin wondering what's left after that. Life might as well be over.

Wrong. Wrong. Wrong.

Let me set the record straight. Life has really just begun. You have a wife and family to provide for, and now is the time you must spring into action and take care of them. By doing so your testosterone levels are not going to decline at the same rate as those individuals who figure life is over.

Your shield of defense against AD will grow larger.

Do not allow depression and irritability to get the best of you, as it will inhibit your ability to provide for your children, spouse, and yourself.

Don't always believe what doctors tell you

Women, too, have the conscious thought that the purpose of their lives is slowly coming to an end as their children start leaving home. The empty nest syndrome envelops them, and they feel deserted and unneeded.

Well, again, let me help set things straight. Your children might be leaving home physically but emotionally you are very much needed. And, if you let depression or irritability set in, you will not be able to guide your children through one of their most vulnerable periods of life as they enter a most hostile society on their own. You have already gained knowledge from the same experience. Pass that knowledge on.

Both you and I have heard parents say, "They only call when they need something." But isn't that statement proof in itself that those parents are, indeed, still very much needed? Think of it in a positive light and the time that passes between phone calls won't seem as long as it did before.

My wife Sandy and I were devastated when a girl we had hoped to adopt was taken from us. When that happened my testosterone level dropped like a rock. Where I had not done so before, I suddenly suffered all the symptoms of male menopause. But through commonsense approaches including proper diet those symptoms began to subside until they were all gone.

Doctors diagnosed Sandy as going through menopause. But I proved them wrong. While I was writing this book, Sandy became pregnant. She is happy again. Her purpose in life is back and all the symptoms of menopause are gone.

Who says that you can't reverse menopause and restart production and secretion of testosterone and estrogen?

Sandy and I are proof that it is possible.

Cortisol: the death hormone

Have you ever wondered why your doctor will only give you cortisone in limited quantities and only for a short period of time? (Cortisone is the drug doctors prescribe. Cortisol is what your body produces.)

In high amounts cortisol is very harmful to the mind. Many medical people call it the death hormone. It is definitely a hormone to handle carefully.

You don't have to go to the doctor to increase your cortisol level. It is produced in the adrenal gland; however, how it gets secreted into the bloodstream is under your control.

Cortisol in balanced amounts is very helpful in maintaining body function, and is essential in preparing you to deal with any approaching threat whether it is physical or psychological. It helps prepare your body to fight or take flight. (More on that in a later chapter.)

Stress resulting from any internal or external thought that triggers the fight or flight mechanism increases the cortisol level. It was once believed that after the threat was over the cortisol level would return to normal. This has been proved to be untrue, especially in today's society in which we suppress one stress after another. This process leads to a continuing accumulation of cortisol.

Cortisol and other stress hormones quickly divert blood glucose to muscles so they can be exercised in preparation for the anticipated fight or flight. This cuts down on the amount of glucose available to the Hippocampus, making it easier for cell degeneration to take place. The Hippocampus is ultra sensitive to cortisol and faced with high, continuous building amounts of cortisol, will accelerate the degeneration process.

A lethal chain reaction can be set in motion. Neuron loss (cell death) gradually increases and the immune system goes on hold. Negative plasticity, as described in the previous chapter, begins to occur at a faster pace. When the immune system shuts down, the elimination of beta amyloid ceases. This means that beta amyloid can increase, eventually reaching the stage where it can run amok. Memory cells are literally slaughtered. And AD is often the result.

Melatonin is one of the good guys

As we discussed in Chapter Four, an appropriate amount of sleep is essential. And the hormone melatonin is a very important factor in building a defense against AD.

Melatonin is regulated by light and is most active while one is asleep. But its benefits have just recently begun to be discovered. Maintaining sleep for at least eight hours is essential so that melatonin can carry out its task of helping restore energy to the brain.

As one ages, melatonin levels decline.

Happiness and joy raise serotonin levels. Since melatonin is derived from serotonin, wouldn't it make sense that by enjoying pleasurable stimulants you would not only be raising serotonin levels, but also levels of melatonin?

Melatonin produces arigisinine vascotin, which has an inhibiting effect on cortisol and also neutralizes the body's most toxic free radical, the hydroxyl radical.

As simple as it sounds, it is very true: You can increase the amount of melatonin in your body by increasing joyful experiences in your life.

Why is insulin so important?

Controlling insulin, I believe, is a key factor in the prevention of AD. Much credit needs to be given Barry Sears, Ph.D., author of the book, *THE ZONE*. He does a great service in showing the effects that insulin has on the brain, and how vital it is to maintain a balance between insulin and glucose (which is the brain's only form of nutrition).

Over the last three decades diets rich in carbohydrates have become the norm. The result is that insulin levels have risen dramatically on average.

As insulin levels increase, the body reacts by storing glucose in the liver and muscle cells. Which is fine if you are preparing to run a marathon. But so often you're just sitting in a chair as the glucose in your blood stream is diverted to the liver and muscle cells. This process deprives the brain of glucose and, being its only form of nutrition, the brain starts to falter.

Times this, times thirty years or more and you are pointing yourself toward AD. When you deprive yourself of nutrients the body slowly deteriorates and withers away. So do the brain cells. It's just that you don't notice until it is too late.

I could go on and on talking about the effects of these hard-working hormones and how one is dependent upon the others. But I think you get the idea that balance is the key. Maintain balance with pleasurable stimuli and an energizing diet, and you will be much better able to maintain hormonal balance, greatly increasing the size of your defensive shield against AD.

Chapter Nine: Key points to remember

Testosterone and estrogen are hormones very important to development of the brain.

Conscious thoughts of defeat and loss of purpose in society can bring on menopause in men as well as in women.

Cortisol is produced in the adrenal gland; however, you can control its secretion into your bloodstream and maintain hormonal balance.

You can increase the amount of melatonin in your body by increasing joyful experiences in your life.

Controlling insulin is a key factor in preventing AD.

"Knowledge is power."

Thomas Hobbs

Chapter 10: Don't let genes worry you

As you read this chapter, keep in mind that knowledge is power.

We can't go back in time and change the genes that we inherited from our parents who, in turn, inherited them from their parents, and so on. However, if we know what those genes are, we can use that knowledge to our benefit in building our shield of defense against AD and other diseases.

Success of the Human Genome Project in mapping out our genes has opened the door to positive possibilities that would have been considered science fiction only a few years ago.

Yes, the HGP also has potential for major negative possibilities, such as opening a Pandora's box overflowing with new drugs that will alter genes without eliminating the many causes that lead to disease.

My hope is that common sense will prevail, and that the doors opened as a result of the HGP will be used to develop drug-free avenues that lead to prevention rather than just more never-ending treatments that enrich the coffers of the drug moguls.

Step right up; take the test

On the positive side, the HGP is paving the way for inexpensive tests to determine one's vulnerability to Alzheimer's Disease. You need not fear being tested for what type of ApoE gene or genes you have inherited.

There's been much publicity about the ApoE4 gene that is believed to increase one's odds of getting AD. Don't let what you've read get you down.

Actually, there are three variations of ApoE:

1. ApoE4 which increases one's chances of getting AD

2. ApoE3 which is the most common and, therefore, probably the parent gene

3. ApoE2 which seems to be protective and reduces the risk of AD

Having inherited one gene from each parent, you could have any combination. But there is good news. By knowing your vulnerability to AD, you can adjust your lifestyle and bolster your defense against AD.

We need to know the triggers

When you think about it, doesn't it seem odd that only recent generations of families carrying the ApoE4 gene have been hit hard by AD?

This tells me, as a commonsense researcher, that there must be external triggers that set the stage for the "great mind-robber." We discussed several of those causative factors in Chapter Two.

Also, having based my research on commonsense approaches, I consider the following statistical comparison to be indicative of a crime in progress. By far, most research focuses on the estimated ten percent of AD that is considered familial, meaning that it is inherited. The other ninety percent of people who develop AD have what doctors call sporadic type Alzheimer's, meaning that it could be the result of any number of unknown causes.

Why is very little research being done to find out what causes the ninety percent to contract AD?

Could it be that many billions of dollars can be made through development of unnatural substances that can alter genes?

In a society that has allowed the poison of aspartame to be spread about unchecked, greedy CEOs will continue to develop means of making money at the expense of integrity and the health of the people who buy their products.

There are no "official" statistics to back me up, but I believe that, if greed is not already the No. One cause of unnatural death in the United States, it soon will be.

Sorry about getting up on my soapbox again. Actually, I'm not sorry, because the truth needs to be told.

You can help speed much-needed AD research

Please participate in the questionnaire that comprises most of this book's last chapter. Learning about peoples' backgrounds, lifestyles, and external stimulants will be of great help to me and other researchers dedicated to pinpointing exact causes of AD.

Dr. Alzheimer, nearly a century ago, identified the results of AD by doing an autopsy of a victim's brain. He did not know what factors combined to create the tangles and plaques he had discovered.

What leads to AD in one person might not be what triggers it in another person. By means of massive numbers of people providing answers to specific questions, we can really jump-start the process of identifying and then isolating definite triggers.

With the answers we can help you and your loved ones make the lifestyle changes necessary to delay or prevent the onset of AD. Whether it is a matter of delaying or preventing will depend on how much or how little damage has been triggered in your brain.

Three major factors

PAD is an acronym for three of the major factors that have been studied as to their helpfulness or risk in relation to AD.

1. Physical activity

2. Arteriosclerosis

3. Diabetes

Just using common sense you've already figured out which of the three can be very beneficial, and which two elevate the risk of AD.

Physical activity

Studies have shown that regular physical activity helps ward off AD. Those who carry the ApoE4 gene should find methods of enjoying physical activity on an even more consistent basis than those with ApoE3 or ApoE2 genes

You don't have to suddenly become a hard-core physical fitness nut and possibly risk injuries that will defeat your purpose. Just use some common sense. Some people find methods of enjoyable exercise through jobs that require physical activity. Others who sit behind desks all day might consider scheduling meetings at the golf course or health club. I know one person who walks up and down several flights of stairs during work breaks.

Coach a children's or adult recreational sports team; take the family on regular weekend physical activities in season, such as skiing, hiking, tennis, or swimming.

You get the picture.

There are many things you can do and not inhibit your life in any way, as so many people think.

Physical activity on an ongoing basis lowers cortisol levels. The adrenal gland secretes cortisol in response to stress that our society is so good at producing. We'll talk more about that later.

Arteriosclerosis is a bad guy

In preventing AD, the brain is dependent on the bloodstream to carry the necessary nutrients, chemicals, and hormones from other parts of the body. When one's blood flow is inhibited by the formation of plaques caused by high cholesterol levels over years of accumulation, the brain is not going to get the nutrients, chemicals, and hormones to function properly.

Arteriosclerosis has been found to increase the risk of AD in those carrying the ApoE4 gene. Which is interesting, because ApoE4 has been implicated in the development of arteriosclerosis. ApoE4 gene carriers often have higher levels of cholesterol.

But through a genetic diet one can control cholesterol levels. A strong network of family and friends, as illustrated by the California-Japan study discussed in Chapter Four, also is helpful in lowering the possibility of heart disease and other complications.

Diabetes increases risk of AD

This is especially true for those with the ApoE4 gene. Avoiding diabetes is important; however, if you are diabetic, you can improve your health dramatically with proper diet (as we will discuss in the next chapter) and lifestyle changes including regular exercise.

Insulin helps control glucose, the brain's only form of nutrition. And maintaining balance is critical. Which brings to mind some serious concerns I have about the methods of the American Diabetes Association.

For years this association has recommended a high carbohydrate diet and substituting aspartame for sugar.

Is it the diabetes that is causing increased risk of AD?

Or is it the high carbohydrate diet and the aspartame?

A friend, who was diagnosed in 1997 as being diabetic, suggests that an apt name for the organization might be the American Disabling Association. He is absolutely convinced that a strong case could be made that the recommendations of the ADA not only do not help lessen the complications of diabetes but, on the contrary, assure that the complications will gradually worsen.

If you think I get on my soapbox, you should hear this guy express his opinions about the ADA and where that association gets major funding.

High carbohydrates continuously deprive the brain of glucose as it is diverted to muscle and liver cells. And the energy necessary to break down carbohydrates every day robs other areas of the body of much needed energy.

A balanced diet of seven proteins to ten carbs with moderate intake of fats assures the body of the proper building blocks that in turn assure that plasticity takes place properly. This then helps build the immune system so that it will respond correctly.

Diabetes inhibits the body in many ways, including facilitating arteriosclerosis and disrupting the liver's ability to remove toxins.

What are you going to do regarding testing?

When those inexpensive tests to determine AD and other disease risks are available, are you going to step right up and be tested?

Beside yourself you have a family to be concerned about. As a carrier you pass your genes on to your child like they were passed down to you. And you control your child's first eighteen years of life as we discussed in Chapter Three.

AD is a lifetime progressive disease that can be linked to childhood. But, if you still fear being tested, at least use common sense. Observe others around you, especially elderly family members and relatives. Compare their lives to others. Compare their vulnerabilities to disease to their lifestyles. You can learn from their mistakes rather than from your own, because if you have to learn from your mistakes, it probably will be too late.

It all comes back to plasticity

As learned in previous chapters, plasticity can be good, and it can be bad. Plasticity consists of building and rebuilding neuro networks; also, transporting cholesterol around the central nervous system and in the bloodstream.

One of the functions of ApoE is regulating the assembly and disassembly of microtubules within the neurons. Like the bloodstream, the microtubules are responsible for carrying substances vital for neuron survival. Within these substances are chemicals necessary to prevent mutation of DNA.

But a problem exists for those who carry the ApoE4 gene. Tau cannot bind to the microtubules, inhibiting structural integrity. With such weakened microtubules it is more likely that they will twist and inhibit the mitochondria from receiving the proper levels of chemicals to assure survival.

Mitochondria's main role is energy production. Without energy the neuron cannot survive, and takes the path of degeneration and eventually apopotosis. The resulting cell death increases the accumulation of beta amyloid.

With less stable microtubules it is essential that more repetitive stimulus be received to assure that the mitochondria receives that occasional charge to prevent mutation and the secretion of excess beta amyloid.

I guess what I'm trying to say in these last few paragraphs is simply that a happy and healthy neuron is an excited neuron. So keep them excited as much and as often as you possibly can.

Meanwhile, remember that knowledge is power.

Chapter Ten: Key points to remember

Knowing which ApoE gene or ApoE gene combination you have, will give you power to fend off AD by appropriate changes in diet and exercise.

What leads to AD in one person might not be what triggers it in another person. Which is why it is so important to participate in the questionnaire in Chapter Nineteen.

Physical activity is very beneficial in reducing the risk of AD.

Arteriosclerosis and diabetes elevate the risk of AD.

Take advantage of inexpensive testing that eventually will be made possible by the Human Genome Project.

"The only way to keep your health is to eat what you don't want, drink what you don't like and do what you'd rather not."

Mark Twain

"One cannot think well, love well, sleep well, if one has not dined well."

Virginia Woolf

Chapter 11: Diet for good health & prevention

By the time you have read this chapter I want this acronym for the word diet seared into your memory:

Do

It

Every

Time

One of the best ways to defend against AD and most diseases is to eat a balanced diet. But for it to be continuously effective, **Do It Every Time.**

There is no way I could overestimate the worth of a properly balanced diet. To me this would be an impossible task. Because I've seen first hand far too many times what poor diet does to people of all ages.

Let's put it this way:

Picture a football field between two bleacher stadiums. Two thousand spectators are sitting in the bleacher seats on each side of the field. The spectators on one side have grown up with a habit of regularly eating balanced meals. They've always shunned products with aspartame like the plague. While the fans across the field believe that the word diet only means to starve yourself silly to lose weight. They eat and drink whatever they want whenever they want, and they don't believe that product labels are for reading. They think that if a product is advertised to have aspartame in it, then that's the only diet aid for them. I mean…if it's on TV, it must be true. Right?

Now for the big question:

In which bleacher stadium are the two thousand people that are nearly ninety percent less likely to ever get AD?

You know the answer. If you don't, you've been reading this book with your eyes and mind closed.

Just for the record

The power of advertising has been pretty strong over the last thirty years. How else could you explain the fact that when the vast majority of people today hear the word diet, the first thing they think of is weight loss?

I've never seen the words weight loss in a dictionary definition for diet. On the contrary, diet is defined as one's usual food and drink intake or a regulated selection of food.

What you eat and drink every day is your diet.

Your diet can be regular, irregular, balanced, or unbalanced. It can be just about anything you want it to be. And the key words here are "anything you want it to be."

What is your diet?

Whether it is beneficial or destructive, it is the result of choices that you have made. Hopefully, you've made consistently good choices. This book is all about making good choices. I can't make choices for you; however, I can put leaves of truth out there for you to pick. If I come across as harsh at times it is because that is sometimes the only way I can penetrate the deep skulls that so many people I come in contact with have developed.

Where have consistent diets gone?

We can't just reach out and reclaim all the positives of the past. But it is good to study habits and routines of our parents and their parents, especially before the decade of the '70s.

In the past consistent diets were more often the norm than not. Our diets were very well regulated, with family members sitting down for three square meals a day. Throughout the week foods varied and one received all the nutrients to maintain balance.

Dad was the provider assuring food and shelter. Mom was the doctor nurturing your every need. She prescribed and prepared the necessary meals so that your body got the nutrients it needed. The nutrients were then converted into the proper chemicals to assure full bodily function.

People didn't worry about the word diet, as it was a routine part of their lives. But that is not so true today. Meals are sporadic and the balanced diet has gone the way of vinyl records.

We live in the nuke 'm age of the microwave.

Have you ever wondered, when you go to buy a used home, why the stove always looks so new? Well, it has rarely been used more than once a month.

Then you inspect the rest of the house and observe that the homeowners' children are bouncing off the walls. It's probably because of the bad diet due, in part, to not using the stove. Nuke 'm this, nuke 'm that; save some time right now, save some more time at the next visit to the microwave.

Well, put this thought in your head and let it percolate:

Would you rather save time now and shorten your lifespan?

Or fix properly balanced meals now and live longer with a healthier lifestyle?

Constant state of confusion

The diet industry has grown into a mega-billion-dollar annual business, and the food industry as a whole is into the trillions.

So whom do you listen to?

The folks that are trying to fatten you up by selling you their products?

Or, the ones trying to get you to slim down with theirs?

Stuck in the middle is the F.D.A. That agency has neither the time nor the funding to conduct the necessary studies to keep up with ever-increasing changes coming at it. The result is that the F.D.A. depends on studies done by the product makers themselves.

Do you think that after spending $10,000,000 on research that a company's head honchos are truly going to criticize themselves, as they add patentable synthetic chemicals to the foods we eat?

If so, do I have a deal for you: the Brooklyn Bridge, and this week it's only $9.95.

Advice and a comparison

There was a time when most people, when asked the question, "Whom do you trust the most?" would say Mom and Dad. That's because parents did not have a profit motive to steer their kids wrong. They really did have their children's best interests at heart. They usually meted out good advice to their offspring. And what's intriguing is that often the advice was taken.

How times have changed.

We've lapsed from a lean-and-mean national attitude to one that ignores the obvious increase in obesity, ADHD, immune deficiencies disease, and psychological disorders. All of these conditions used to be rare. And where they did exist, most of the time it involved situations where divorce was splitting family loyalties, or simply because a family was generally dysfunctional, usually as a result of not getting those three square meals a day.

By comparison, Dr. Barry Sears' *The Zone* offers the closest to those diets of the '50s and '60s when AD was still rare. The ratio of seven proteins to ten carbohydrates is similar, with the main difference being the consumption of fats was much higher in those earlier decades.

Fat is another one of those falsely associated words. Fats will make you fat being not necessarily true. We will discuss that later.

Meanwhile, consider again the acronym for diet:

Do

It

Every

Time

Of course, you know by reading this far that a balanced diet works best in association with proper balance in the areas of sleep, physical activity, and pleasure.

Did I mention that you should **Do It Every Time?**

Okay. Okay. I admit that it is not possible to have perfect balance in all areas every day; however, setting that achievement as a daily goal will keep you in the **Zone** as Dr. Sears calls it. Living in the **Zone** is how I regained my health. My advice is that you consider **Zone** living, too.

Maintain that 7-10 ratio

The ratio of foods that we eat controls balance in our daily diet.

Carbohydrates assure the body of glucose, the brain's only form of nutrition.

Proteins are the basis of all life and are the second most abundant substances in our bodies.

Fats assure "essential" fatty acids that are not made by the body.

So what went wrong?

For three decades we have been hammered with advice to consume high carbohydrates and little or no fats. Proteins have been downplayed.

Now, at the other end of those decades, obesity among adults and children is at an all-time high. Our population on average can barely defeat the common cold and disease is increasing every year.

For whose best interests were these diets developed?

Could it be the manufacturers of highly profitable carbohydrates?

Or the medical and drug industries that reap enormous profits in repairing the damage caused during the previous thirty years?

What's been foisted on us is truly not in our best interest. And when that rare event happens when a company actually admits a misdeed, the best we usually get is an, "Oops! We've made a mistake. Give us ten or twenty more years to complete the research and conduct our studies, and we'll get back with you."

Let's hear it for proteins

Proteins are made up of amino acids. Of the twenty-two known amino acids eight are essential and must be brought into the body in the foods we eat to assure the proper building of all proteins.

Proteins are necessary in the creation of new neurons as positive plasticity takes place; also, in the removal of unwanted and unneeded neurons during the process of negative plasticity.

A 7 protein to 10-carbohydrate ratio is essential to create and maintain hormonal balance. But precautions must be taken because, along with protein intake comes high levels of saturated fats. Eating leaner cuts of meat will help lower those levels.

To avoid meats containing antibiotics, growth-inducing hormones, pesticides, and herbicides that come down the food chain, my dad used to buy beef quarters and halves from stock raised by kids involved with 4H activities. It was great-tasting beef.

Go easy on those carbs

Carbohydrates are made of simple sugars and supply the body with energy. Sugar, fruit, and vegetables all add to the carbs count. Now that you know this, why not stop pouring tons of sugar on that bowl of cereal in the morning to get that quick fix?

When one stays close to that 7 to 10 ratio all is fine and the body, including the brain, works in harmony. The proteins are then enabled to do their building to facilitate plasticity, and the right amount of carbs will assure appropriate energy.

As the body converts carbs to glucose the resulting glucose is used up as a source of energy. But as that conversion takes place the body has limited storage capacity for glucose. Once the energy needs are met and storage capacity filled, carbs are then converted into fats. It is a six-hour cycle that is always taking place.

By limiting carbohydrate intake to a 7 to 10 ration, one will get all the energy that is necessary for the body to function properly on an ongoing basis.

Increasing your carbohydrate intake, as so many people do, will throw the body out of balance.

Remember when you ate that first bag of potato chips and you couldn't eat just one – even if you tried to hold back? Well, the manufacturers latched on to that idea to sell more of their products. A vicious, but very profitable cycle was created. Eating too many carbs threw the body out of balance. Then followed a process of eating more products to try and bring the body back into balance; and then eating even more products, compounding the situation.

The ad campaigns have been working. We consume more carbohydrates than ever before.

The mind becomes a glucose hog with its demands for more glucose to carry out the tasks of thought and plasticity. The quick fix is to increase carb and sugar intake; however, as we discussed in Chapter Nine, a problem arises with insulin, so necessary in glucose control. Once the body meets its glucose need, insulin signals the liver and muscle cells to store the excess glucose.

As insulin levels increase, blood-glucose levels decrease thereby robbing the brain of much needed energy. What usually happens next is that more carbs are quickly consumed, so on ad infinitum. Trying to keep glucose in balance with such high levels of carbs overtaxes the pancreas (which produces insulin) to the point where it becomes worn out and around age fifty, diabetes is diagnosed.

If you absolutely must have those high levels of carbs, at least increase your physical activity. That will help the body in maintaining balance.

Much energy is needed to break down carbs, which in turn robs energy from the brain and the immune system. Energy is lost that otherwise would have been used for plasticity and maintaining a proper immune response in eliminating beta amyloid before it is allowed to accumulate.

The key to carbs control is to consume just enough of them to supply the body with energy on an ongoing basis. If within a half-hour after consuming a meal you feel bogged down and have an urge to grab more carbs to perk you up, you know that you took in too many carbs at the last meal and have thrown your body out of balance.

It is not easy to get out of cycles that have become strong habits, but once one does, the resulting feeling of balance will be enjoyed as energy and desires to do things start to return. Along the road to balance a lot of those little aches and pains will go away.

Now for that discussion about fats

Fats do not produce fat if consumed correctly. One of the major reasons for obesity is high carb intake. Once the body is supplied with the energy it needs and storage capacity filled, carbs are converted into fat.

Fat is essential in one's diet to maintain proper body function. Per gram, fats provide twice the number of calories as do carbohydrates or protein, and are important as an energy source.

Energy-supplying carbs are usually burned up during the first twenty minutes of exercise, and then the body begins to depend on calories from fats to provide energy.

In modest amounts fat is very beneficial. Fats provide the essential fatty acids that are not made by the body and must be consumed. The membranes of neurons are made up of fats and supply the neurons with the essential fats that must be consumed to assure that positive plasticity takes place in the formation of new neurons.

A child from birth to two years old is never put on a low fat diet as fat is so essential for growth and development, especially in regard to the brain.

Although growth stops in early adulthood, the body is constantly repairing and rebuilding itself. This has been known for years. While the discovery by scientists that the mind, too, is continually rebuilding itself as plasticity takes place was only made in the last decade.

The brain demands fat to facilitate plasticity. Deprive the body of essential fats that must be consumed and you are denying the body the building blocks necessary in the production of new neurons through neurogenesis.

And those hormones and neurotransmitters so important in full body function are highly dependent on fats.

Every steroid, which includes estrogen, is made from cholesterol. Yet in the last thirty years we've been told to avoid cholesterol. Now they're saying avoid only the bad cholesterol. Well, you need both in modest amounts to assure proper body and brain function.

I could go on forever describing how an unbalanced died creates imbalance with the body. But I think you get the idea. If nothing else, you've learned a good acronym for diet: **Do It Every Time.**

Chapter Eleven: Key points to remember

A balanced diet is one of the best defenses against AD and other diseases.

Read Dr. Barry Sears' book, *The Zone*.

Maintain a 7-10 ratio of proteins to carbohydrates.

Fats do not produce fat if consumed correctly.

A good acronym for DIET is:

Do

It

Every

Time

Keep all your meals balanced.

"I like nonsense; it wakes up the brain cells."

Dr. Seuss

"The human race has one really effective weapon, and that is laughter."

Mark Twain

Chapter 12: Paying attention & pleasure pay big time

What would you do if your doctor diagnosed you as being terminally ill and told you that, at best, you had six more months to live?

Well, if you were Norman Cousins, you would turn to laughter as the best medicine.

When Cousins was first given that news, of course he had an emotional letdown; however, he did not give up, lie down, and wait to die. He looked inside himself and examined what he saw: negative influences including anger, worry, and depression had affected his health.

Ok, he reasoned, if negativity could make his health bad, couldn't positive activity help him become well again?

Cousins resolved to make of his self a one-person experiment. He rented all the movie comedies he could find. No, he didn't have the luxury of simply going to a video rental outlet, because that was before the VCR. What he rented were actual films.

He discovered that by laughing continuously for five minutes the intense, relentless pain that inflicted him would ease off enough for him to get several hours' sleep. His appetite for laughter grew. His friends read and told him stories that kept his laughter flowing.

Yes. Norman Cousins laughed himself to good health. He lived for another twenty happy, productive years. He wrote the book *Anatomy of an Illness* in which he credited visualization, love of family and friends, and healing laughter for his recovery.

You can't underestimate positive pleasure

What a powerful example Cousins set for us all. Here is how I would briefly outline his experiment:

1. He searched for and found the problem.

2. He developed a plan of positive action.

3. He kept his focus on that plan.

4. He got positive results.

Or, put another way, Cousins set a goal to achieve good health, visualized good health, and achieved good health.

More simply put, he made a decision to do something, and then he followed through and did it.

What decisions do you need to make?

Some are easy. Others are hard to make. You have to weigh the benefits of putting feet under your decisions. Can you visualize those benefits as reality? Are those benefits worth striving for?

Or, as a friend would put it, are you a man or a mouse, a woman or a worm?

It's an epic battle: stress vs. pleasure

We live in a complex society fueled by stress. Stress is inevitable. It's here to stay. Our economy is based on it, and through the passing of stress from one individual to another, our economy has thrived.

Our ancestors survived much stress as they went through WWI, the Great Depression, and then into WWII. They went through periods lasting years at a time with no immediate relief in sight. Many of them are still around to tell their tales.

Stress today sets the population up for unending disease possibilities. But that was often not the case with our ancestors.

Why not?

It is because they maintained thoughts of pleasure. The anticipation of victory and believing they would return to their families gave them a sense of pleasure and greatly increased their testosterone levels.

Talk to holocaust victims and they will tell you that continuous thoughts of being reunited with family and friends kept their hopes up during the tragic times they lived through. They were balancing stress with pleasure. And it worked as very few holocaust survivors suffered from early onset of AD.

We've forgotten what worked in the past

Today the power of pleasure to balance one's hormones is very much under used, and the power of family unification is becoming extinct.

No longer do people work for forty years and then spend their savings on an enjoyable retirement. Instead, they pass their savings on to the medical and drug industries thereby creating even more stress as their savings dwindle away.

All of this can easily be turned around if you latch on to the power of pleasure and family cohesiveness like your ancestors did to assure their survival.

My grandfather, a WWI veteran who passed away only a few years ago, enjoyed a life free of disease. From him I learned the power of a united family. His life goals were simple: fulfill the needs of his children as his parents had fulfilled his, and hoping the process would be repeated in my generation with my parents fulfilling my needs. Those goals were met.

Learn the art of balancing

Putting and keeping balance in your life goes beyond your diet, physical activity, and nurturing. It includes balancing stress and pleasure, the latter being perhaps the most powerful tool in preventing disease.

Like a high carbohydrate diet, stress diverts glucose to muscles preparing you to fight or take flight, further robbing the brain of glucose (it's only form of nutrition).

But unlike what happens with high carb intake, cortisol is secreted from the adrenal gland isolating the neuron cells in the hippocampus. This puts reasonable thought and the immune system on hold. All the while one might just be sitting at an office desk getting chewed out by his boss or be at home just worrying about the bills that need to be paid.

If no physical activity takes place to use the stress hormones that have prepared your body to fight or take flight, those hormones start to accumulate from one stressful situation to another, causing continuous isolation of the neuron cells within the hippocampus. The immune system is further shut down, inhibiting the removal of beta amyloid.

Stress unavoidable, balance still possible

Yes, that is a true statement. Even though stress is unavoidable, one can balance one's hormones with pleasure.

In medical terms, stress excites the sympathetic nervous system (SNS) and the cholinergic pathway (acetycholine neurotransmitter). Pleasure excites the parasympathetic nervous system (PNS) and the dopaminergic pathway (dopamine neurotransmitter).

One wants to seek balance by exciting the PNS, as this will activate a relaxation response that will reestablish homeostasis (balance). Included in the response are elevated seretonin levels that will increase melatonin, which, in turn, will inhibit cortisol.

The hydroxyl free radical will then be removed by melatonin's by-product, argisimine vascotocin.

Result: the odds of preventing AD and lowering cortisol levels are greatly enhanced.

In layman terms, there are many beneficial hormones and neurotransmitters secreted when you are enjoying pleasurable activities. So, enough of the medical terminology as it is quite complicated and confusing.

So, how do I get that balance?

It is relatively easy to achieve. Remember the example of the Wednesday night outing previously discussed involving a 24-hour hotel/motel room rental?

Well, that is one of the methods that will help bring you back into balance.

In the job you have, does your employer give you time to at least communicate with your family during working hours? If not, consider moving on. At the time of this writing, we're in a strong economy, and many other jobs are available (if you just look). Many corporations are family friendly and, as a result, enjoy much larger profit margins and growth than do their dominating employer rivals. Microsoft has proved that.

That little note in the lunch box will give your child that much-needed boost during the middle of the day.

And a love letter to your spouse via e-mail at lunchtime will do the same. Not to mention the positive side effects you will benefit from when you get home.

Nature has given us time for balance: eight hours of stress (job), eight hours of pleasure, and eight hours of sleep, with a forty-eight-hour margin (weekend) thrown in for good measure.

What more could we ask for?

How one interprets the meaning of stress or pleasure is very widespread in our society. Only you can set your levels of stimulus to create balance. Far too many people consider family as stressful and jobs as pleasure. This is a trend that needs to be reversed. With time and passion it can easily be done to assure that the whole family – not just one's self – can achieve balance.

Decisions need to be made.

Remember that three-hours-per-day concept we discussed in Chapter Three? If you have children at home, that would be one of the greatest life investments you could possibly make. And you'd still have ninety-seven percent of your life to do with as you wish.

Pay attention, do it often

I don't want to hear, "Well, I don't have the time."

All it involves is shifting a little bit of time and paying attention to others on a more consistent basis. How long does it take to pick up a phone and call just to tell someone that you care and that you miss that person and will be in touch soon? Two minutes! So what's the big deal? Take advantage of the vast network of communications technology that exists today.

Whether mate to mate, parent to children, or vice versa, it's not so important what you do together as it is that you are both receiving and showing attention together.

More and more recent studies are showing that children from large families are more prone to have AD later in life. I strongly believe that the underlying reason for this is primarily one of attention. The more children in a family, the harder it is to provide equal, positive attention to each child. With attention being more divided chances are increased that neuron network growth will be inhibited.

Now, consider children in general in our society. The majority of the little ones are in daycare centers were personnel have to divide their attention amongst five babies and toddlers from birth to age two; then amongst ten kids from age two until preschool; then, when they go to school, a teacher's attention is usually spread over meeting the needs of twenty to thirty children.

What a tragic formula. No wonder children today have trouble defeating the common cold. They probably retained only one-fourth of the neurons and connections they were born with, instead of the fifty percent that is considered normal retention at age three.

It's all largely due to lack of attention. And a lot of moms and dads sure aren't going to make up the difference after coming home from work exhausted.

A most interesting stress study

When researchers on the payroll of drug companies do trial studies on the safety of drugs and food additives, they do so under what are considered "ideal conditions." In addition, they almost always take for granted that the drugs or additives they are testing will not pass through what is called the "blood-brain barrier."

This barrier is a self-defense mechanism whereby the brain bars molecules of foreign substances from actually entering the brain and doing damage. A lot of drugs and additives are sold that would, indeed, do much harm should they penetrate that barrier and run amok inside the brain.

Using the existence of this barrier as an excuse, many manufacturers claim that there is no need to worry that their toxic products will pass through the blood-brain barrier. This might be true under ideal conditions. But when was the last time you've seen ideal conditions in this complex society?

During the Gulf War, Israeli soldiers were given a drug called pyridostigmine for protection against chemical and biological weapons. About one-fourth of them complained of headaches, nausea, and dizziness. Those symptoms occur only if the drug enters the brain.

So why had the side effects increased during combat? That question led an Israeli biochemist and a physician to consider that the stress of war had allowed molecules of the drug to pass through the blood-brain barrier. The test study they came up with involved a group of mice, some of which were stressed by dunking them in water. Dye was injected into the mice. Brain autopsies showed much higher concentrations of dye inside the brains of the stressed animals.

Conclusion: stress can dramatically increase the ability of chemicals to pass through the blood-brain barrier.

Just thinking about what the medical and drug communities have foisted on us as being safe is cause for stress. I'm ready to watch a funny movie. How about you?

Chapter Twelve: Key points to remember

Sometimes laughter really is the best medicine.

Even though stress is unavoidable, you can balance your hormones with pleasure.

Stress can enable dangerous drugs to penetrate the blood-brain barrier and disrupt and even destroy hormonal balance.

Paying attention to others can be just as important as pleasure in building up your defenses against disease.

"A woman never gets too old not to be held in a man's arms."

68-year-young woman

Chapter 13: Human touch saves lives

Remember when you first heard the story about King Midas? You probably wished that you, too, could turn everything into gold that you touched. At least, you had that desire until you heard the rest of the story.

When the greedy king's cat brushed up against his leg, the feline instantly became a golden statute. The same thing happened when the king's daughter rushed in and started to kiss and hug her father.

He couldn't even toss a grape into his mouth without it turning into gold. When he tried to take a drink, goblet and liquid also were transformed.

What to do? What to do?

He knew that he would die of thirst and starvation if his golden touch were not taken from him. After promising that he would not be greedy anymore, he was told what to do so that he, his cat, and daughter could be reunited in living flesh.

More valuable than gold

Human touch is far more valuable than gold as it can save lives rather than destroy them. Appropriate, caring, loving touch is like a bottled-up miracle available to anyone willing to pour out its healing powers.

Many studies have confirmed the positive power of touch, and also the negative power of withholding touch.

Consider the experiment of real-life Frederick II, Holy Roman emperor and king of Southern Italy. Back in the 13th century he came up with the notion that babies might have an "inborn" language and he wanted to discover it. He ordered that a group of babies be raised that were never to be spoken to by their mothers or nursemaids.

Even though the basic physical needs, i.e., food and drink, were met, most of the babies died. Frederick II was surprised by the results. He did not know that babies need emotional connective ness with their mothers via touch and baby talk.

Attachment is critical to physical and neurological development of children. The severing of that bond causes negative changes in heart rate, immune response, and stress hormones.

What about more recent studies?

Psychiatrist Rene Spitz conducted a famous study in the 1940s. She made comparisons involving two groups of babies. One group was raised in a home for babies that had been abandoned or orphaned. The other group consisted of infants raised in a nursery accessible to their mothers who were in prison.

Both institutions were similar in that they were clean and provided the babies with sufficient food, clothing, and medical care. However, there was a huge difference in the levels of nurturing and stimulation provided.

The imprisoned moms cared for their offspring one-to-one, pouring attention and affection over them. Despite the institution setting, those children developed normally.

By contrast, the infants in the foundling home were subjected to a ratio of one nurse per eight babies. Except for systematic feedings and diaper changes, those babies were isolated in cribs whose sides were draped with sheets to prevent the spread of infection.

Can you imagine what happens to infants who have nothing to play with or look at, and who have a bare minimum of human contact and affection? Many of them did not survive to age two.

The Schanberg, Field study

Dr. Saul Schanberg of Duke University and Tiffany Field of the University of Miami worked first with animals, then with human "preemies." What they found reinforces the tremendous importance of touch.

Preemies routinely were isolated in incubators bearing Do Not Touch signs. As they were so tiny, doctors believed it best that they should not be disturbed, because anything that caused them to cry would endanger their breathing.

The preemies were well fed and their medical needs met; however, most of them did not grow. Many became physically and mentally retarded, or died.

Schanberg and Field found out why through a series of experiments on rats. When they separated newborn rats from their mothers, the pups went into a survival mode. In the process of conserving food and energy, body growth stopped. Stress hormones released to control the hunger urge turned off genetic activity so cells would not divide.

By reuniting the pups with their mothers, the stress hormones abated and normal growth returned.

Through the process of elimination, the scientists found that the mother's licking kept their newborns happy and the stress hormones in balance.

Switching their focus to the preemies, the researchers found the same chemical changes taking place. The major stress hormone cortisol was up and DNA synthesis was down.

Unlike with rat pups, human babies are not licked, but they are held and their backs are rubbed. Schanberg and Field tried that with the preemies, and the infants began to thrive and grow stronger.

The touching and rubbing led to a doubling of growth rates for many of the babies. Average hospital stay was reduced six to seven days as compared to the longer stays required for the "untouched" infants, and at a cost reduction of about $5,000 per baby.

Just another example of what commonsense approaches can accomplish.

Proof up close and personal

Our son Michael, after a very traumatic birth, was placed in an incubator. He was yellow in color and was having problems breathing.

It was only after my wife and I succeeded with our demands to touch and hold him that his color returned to normal and his breathing problems went away never to return.

We learned early on the dramatic effects appropriate touch has on children.

One of our society's sad commentaries is that agenda-seeking people are creating an atmosphere where human touch is bad. Parents, teachers, and society in general fear touching children, afraid that they will be accused of inappropriate touch.

Yet businesses use it every day in the form of a handshake or the casual placing by a salesman of his arm around one's shoulder trying to close a deal on a car sale, hoping to create that bond of trust associated with human touch.

First, starting the process with a child, one must help that young human set up foundational neuron networks that relate human touch to positive and loving events. Creating such foundations is a formidable step toward the prevention of AD. It also will greatly lessen the possibility of that child growing into a teenager who seeks fulfillment through sexual encounters.

A hug and kiss, or just the rubbing of one's back, whether it be a child, grandchild, spouse, or aging parent or grandparent, is so important in life.

Many children have come through my wife's and my life, that are so obviously depleted of the hormones oxytocin and vasopressin. Foster children often have serious hormone deficiencies. Yet the Social Services people instruct you not to touch them.

For the first two months that we cared for foster children, I was very reluctant to touch them. But as time went on and through reading, research, and just through personal experience, I could no longer deny them something so essential to maintain balance in life. I gave out hugs and back rubs. The Social Services people accused me of setting up the children to molest them in the future. We eventually lost these children for doing what even scientific studies have shown to be the right thing to do.

Do it throughout life

Human touch is important throughout one's life, as it stimulates skin cells to start the chain reaction necessary to maintain hormone levels physically and emotion-ally.

For most happily married couples, ultimate touch and pleasure is found through regular sexual intimacy.

Oftentimes divorce results from the lack of positive sexual union, as one or both mates seek out attention from other individuals perceived as caring for them.

No matter how young or old you are, appropriate touch has rejuvenating powers.

As that commercial says, "Reach out and touch someone."

Preferably, someone you love, like your mate, children, parents, or grandparents.

Go ahead. Give it a try.

Chapter Thirteen: Key points to remember

Human touch can save lives.

Appropriate touch has dramatic, positive effects on infants, children, mates, parents, and grandparents.

"Where all men think alike, no man thinks very much."

Walter Lippmann

Chapter 14: Take control of your thought patterns

People who think for their selves are in the minority these days. Which is another sad commentary on our society. It's as if we've become a nation of sheep blindly following most any shepherd that comes along.

Who is telling the truth?

Who is scamming us?

What can I do about it?

For starters, if you are not already doing so on a regular basis, you can learn to think for yourself.

Chances are that, if you've absorbed and thought through what I've thrown at you so far in this book, you already have good thought pattern ability. Should that be the case with you, fantastic! I believe you will learn how to strengthen your thinking powers even more through using the process of cognitive thought.

Not the genes, but the triggers

I hope by now you realize that Alzheimer's Disease is not caused by genes, but how one triggers those genes. Most triggering takes place through conscience thought, the decisions that one makes.

Those who do not take control of their own thoughts and decisions set themselves up for a possible trip down the path to AD. That's the path whose travelers eventually lose the ability to make conscious and reasonable decisions.

Many people we have trusted to steer us down the right paths have steered us wrong. No longer can we depend on others doing our thinking for us. From years of listening, our minds have become very confused as to whom to listen to. We need to take control of our own thoughts and start making reasonable decisions, based on facts, and not on what the so-called experts are telling us.

Which is quite easy to accomplish through cognitive thought therapy. It allows us to become independent thinkers so that we can take and keep control of our lives.

Develop the ability to think twice

Very important in taking control over our lives is the ability to think twice, which in itself has become almost a lost art. Impulses and the desire for that quick fix are already dominating many of our lives.

But, through the process of cognitive thought, thinking twice can become so comfortable that you will begin to do it automatically.

Every situation is influenced by the key factors of desire and consequence. Far too often people get so caught up in the desires of the moment that they try not to even consider what the consequences will be.

For example, do I need that product which is laced with aspartame so that I can get that quick fix, and suffer the consequences later?

Or do I cuddle with my spouse on the couch?

Both choices will result in raising the phynylalanine levels in my blood stream. But cuddling on the couch is also going to raise dopamine, serotonin, oxytocin, and vasopressin, and help in creating hormonal balance.

Which activity will I choose?

If I think twice about it, and consider which choice will be the most beneficial in the long run, I will probably opt for cuddling.

This is just one example of thinking twice, and a very simple one at that. Apply the technique of thinking twice as you reevaluate your diet, relationships, and your life in general. Think twice consistently and down the road you most likely will not have to go to your doctor and have him evaluate your symptoms, then tell you that they indicate AD is on your horizon.

Thinking twice is just using common sense.

A matter of perception

As discussed previously, how one perceives stress or pleasure has an effect on cortisol control.

In today's complex society, we have to take on many tasks at once. No longer do we go to work at 8:00 and leave for home at 5:00. We stress ourselves out thinking about how will we ever get it all done. Our hormones get out of balance and cortisol levels rise. Which is bad.

A lot of working moms wake up with that thought process already in motion: How am I going to get to work on time? I have so much to do. Got to fix breakfast, dress myself, put on make-up, dress the kids, and get them to daycare.

But, you know what?

Each morning it all gets accomplished and all is well when you get to work. But here comes that stress again when the boss throws a stack of papers on your desk and says, "I need it by the end of the day."

And again, somehow, you get it all done and heave a great sigh of relief as you head for your car. As you start driving toward home, here that stress comes again as you worry about the stack of laundry you left that morning, how in the world will it get done, the hoeing that needs to be done, fixing dinner, helping the kids with homework, and paying all the bills so that they don't shut off the electricity, water, or telephone.

Guess what happens?

It all gets done.

So what in the world are you worried about?

Most of us have become experts in completing many tasks at one time. We've proven it for years.

And what should we change?

Our perception.

Start each morning perceiving what needs to be done that day as a way of life, and not as things that will heap more stress upon stress.

View it as a way of life that has given all of us many pleasures that were not enjoyed by our ancestors, and that keeps our economy strong. Once you do perceive it as a way of life and not stress, you will enjoy the benefits of lower cortisol levels.

"Catch 22" – that double-edged sword

Granted, life today is not easy but very complicated. To succeed at it you must walk down the center of that double-edged sword with balance.

And to accomplish balance it takes much thought, as you ask yourself questions: Do I work my tail off to provide luxuries for my family as I've been taught, or do I spend more time with them and delay or forego some of the luxuries?

Our society has transformed into one in which status is based on wealth, and not on happiness or health. People, like lemmings marching over the cliff to their own destruction, latch on to status as something of great importance.

Through clear, conscious thought you can begin to achieve your dreams, but it must start by taking some simple, but very important steps:

Cut down on carbs so your brain can get the glucose it needs for nutrition.

Change your perception of stress to lower cortisol levels and stop the isolation of neurons.

Only then are you going to achieve clear conscience thought and be able to walk down the center of that double-edged sword toward balance.

It's easy through clear thought

We talked earlier about the importance of giving to and receiving attention from others. But how do you do it if you are working all the time?

It's easy through clear thought.

When one is thinking clearly and not impulsively, he or she can think up all kinds of methods for showing and receiving attention, and make a good living at the same time. Many methods are disclosed in this book, so half the battle has been won; you just have to apply them.

Cognitive thought therapy was pioneered in the late 1960s by Philadelphia psychiatrists Aaron Beck M.D. and David Burns M.D. It is based on the simple idea that thoughts and attitudes are not controlled by external events, but by how one perceives those events.

It is not based on the principles of Freud, which are almost a century old. Would you let someone perform surgery on your brain using techniques that never worked well in the first place? Freud was given a chance for several decades, during which time emotional disorders increased almost yearly.

Adaptation to new ideas is usually a slow process. It goes against the grain of those whose ways are set in concrete. Especially when the old ways brought profits into the coffers.

Cognitive therapy offers a drug free solution, which automatically makes it a path that drug companies do not want you to take. Depending on one's ability to change habits, ten to thirty sessions will propel one on to a more pleasurable life.

Exercises to correct distorted thinking

The principles of cognitive thought therapy are simple and consist of exercises designed to correct distorted thinking that elevates cortisol levels.

Gaining or regaining control of your thoughts really can be quite easy if you know your negative thought patterns, and how to control them.

The ten basic forms of distorted thinking are:

"All or nothing" thinking: You take on all the problems at one time, such as laundry, preparing meals, and paying the bills.
Solution: Take on one task at a time, come up with a solution, and move to the next task.

Overgeneralization: Taking a situation such as laundry, preparing meals or paying the bills to the next level so that the dominoes start to fall. Do I have the detergent? What am I going to prepare? And where am I going to get the money to pay the bills?
Solution: Do not build upon negative thoughts.

Mental Filter: Dwelling upon only the negative tasks that you have to perform.
Solution: Upon completion, many of these tasks will bring you much pleasure. You will have clean clothes to wear, you will be full of energy after you eat, the bills will be paid, and you won't receive them for another thirty days.

Discounting the Positive: After finishing tasks you feel unappreciated or unneeded.
Solution: Just think if you weren't there, what a mess it would be. Go ahead, take off for a week, and the rest of the family will come to appreciate all those minute tasks, and show you that you are much needed.

Jumping to Conclusions: You assume on the way to work that your boss is going to load you up with work.
Solution: So be it, that's what work is all about, and if they load you up each day, ask for a raise, and if you don't get it, move on.

Magnification: Example, your child brings home a letter to schedule a teacher conference, and your mind focuses on the reason for it.

Solution: Request a note from the teacher with a brief description of the purpose of the conference. Not all teacher conferences are derogatory.

Emotional reasoning: You think with your emotions. You neglect your tasks just because you are depressed, only to have your tasks start piling up.

Solution: Do not let emotion get in the way of your conscious thought on an ongoing task so you can stop those tasks from accumulating. Stop passing emotions on to others; discuss your problems.

Should and Shouldn't statement: You blame yourself for things that have gone wrong, such as "I should have," or "What if I had done that differently?"

Solution: Not by yourself can you accomplish all the tasks all the time. Things happen; you're human.

Labeling: Each day you say to yourself, "What am I doing? I'm a jerk, a fool, a loser." All just because you made a mistake.

Solution: Here again, you're only human. If you accomplish it just eighty percent of the time, you're doing better than most people in this complicated world.

Personalization and blame: You blame yourself for something that you were not entirely responsible for, or overlooking your own contributions to the problems.

Solution: You are not always to blame as usually you are functioning as a family. We all make mistakes. When you do make a mistake, take responsibility and move on. Guide other family members when they err. Don't criticize yourself or others; just remember that we're all human.

It all sounds so simple, because it is. I know from personal experience that knowing the ten steps and applying the solutions that this is an effective way to lower cortisol levels.

Bigger problems need greater solutions, but the principles remain the same, and if applied, one can conquer almost anything, including preventing the onset of AD.

For more advice on the subject, I highly recommend that you read Dr. Burns' books, *The New Mood Therapy*, and *The Feeling Good Handbook.* You can teach yourself the principles of cognitive thought therapy. And for those stubborn individuals who insist on professional assistance, there are psychologists around that offer cognitive thought therapy.

But precautions need to be taken as this form of therapy still is considered fairly new, even though it was developed way back in the 1960s. Seeking out such psychologists can sometimes be difficult. Don't be afraid to question their training in the field of cognitive thought therapy. If they can't quickly tell you the ten forms of distorted thought, move on, as they are still practicing the principles of Freud.

Chapter Fourteen: Key points to remember

Alzheimer's Disease is not caused by genes, but by how you trigger those genes.

Most triggering takes place through conscious thought, the decisions that you make.

The ability to think twice is just using common sense.

How you perceive stress or pleasure affects cortisol control.

Cognitive thought therapy can correct distorted thinking that elevates cortisol levels.

"As selfishness and complaint pervert and cloud the mind, so sex with its joy clears and sharpens the vision."

Helen Keller

Chapter 15: Go ahead, get physical

How many times, perhaps while watching your children or grandchildren play, have you said, "I wish I had their energy"?

Lately, have you been saying to no one in particular, "My get-up-and-go has got up and gone"?

Or, have you joined the legions of couch potatoes so married to their furniture that they even ask someone else to bring the remote control to them?

Some people are so far out of physical shape that it tires their brains when the word exercise comes up.

Maybe it is not people, but bathroom scales that are under the most pressure these days. This gives a whole new meaning to the phrase "lighten up."

The bottom line in any such discussion is this:

Do you submit your life to "won't power"?

Or, do you control it with "will power"?

Get into the balancing act

We've talked about balancing our hormones, diet, and thought patterns. Now, we'll talk a little bit more about balancing ourselves physically.

Less attention over the past few decades has been given to physical activity. Just look around you. Businesses are turning to automation. The gym is the first thing to go when they cut school budgets, as school administrators claim learning is the priority. (But how can that be when administrative costs take huge chunks out of school budgets, and school curricula are constantly being revised to further dumb down our society?)

More and more wage earners are holding down two jobs, plus the one or two jobs that consume their spouses' schedules.

Whatever happened to the notion of more leisure time?

Or, actually seeing and being with little Johnny as he grows up?

Unless you have a job that requires physical exertion, everyday, normal physical activity is no longer a way of life for much of the population. Heck, many couples have to check their separate calendars just to schedule time when they can both be awake for some intimate moments in bed together.

The fight or flight factor

Remember that fight or flight mechanism that kicks in those stress hormones? Well, they are preparing you for the fight that is about to take place if you have to defend yourself, or to flee if you need to.

Both reactions beg for physical activity, because, without a physical response, cortisol starts to build up.

In today's society, physical fighting and fleeing are not acceptable. We resolve our problems on paper, and the only physical activity that takes place is pushing a pen or dialing the phone to call the appropriate authority so a report can be filled out and filed.

Look for alternatives

As the stress hormones kick in, one must seek alternative methods to burn them up. After each stressful situation, for example, your boss chews you out, go for a walk. Don't take the elevator, but use the stairs. By the time you get to the car you will be back in balance. But if he or she chews you out too often, use the car to go get another job.

There are many alternative ways of getting valuable exercise. I have confidence that you already know several of those ways. But don't just think about using them, and say, "I'll start tomorrow."

It may only be a day away in the musical for Little Orphan Annie; however, for many people one tomorrow leads to two tomorrows, and tomorrow never comes.

To put it bluntly, when you do your final life review, do you want to remember most what could have been, or what you actually did?

Flush those excuses

I hear it now. "Well, I go to the gym twice a week." That's just great! You've won half the battle, but you're not going to win the war.

Cortisol shuts down your immune system, and 100% efficiency is what you seek, not 50%. Adjust your physical activity so that it balances with your stress, and think twice. If you suffer an hour of stress each day, balance it with an hour of physical activity. If you can't find an hour in your busy schedule, find half-an-hour and increase the intensity of the workout. Jog instead of walk.

In the previous chapter, you learned how to use the power of thinking. Use that knowledge and make a habit of maintaining balance on a daily basis.

A precaution to think about

That gym you go to each day, well, that's taking time away from your family, and when you get home you get chewed out again for not being with them, and back up goes your cortisol levels.

Communication is so important. Explain that you go to the gym to cut down your stress hormones created by your job, which creates anger, and you don't want to bring it home with you, adding that you want to do your part in making home a place of pleasure.

Mix it up a little. Go to the gym two nights a week, coach your child's sports team on two nights, and just take a pleasurable walk with your spouse on the other nights.

Walk the mall if need be, and spend the money that you save from not having to go to the psychologist or doctor so often.

If you can't meet the goals of balance during the week, make good use of the weekend to create that balance before you start all over on Monday at that stressful job.

There are a lot of ways to prevent muscle melt daily, even while you are at work. For example, you can use isometric exercise to maintain muscle tone. This means simple muscle contraction like results when you suck in your gut and tense your chest muscles while holding your breath for a few seconds as you repeat the process several times. Just clenching your fists in repetitive sets can tone up hand, wrist and arm muscle.

Creating resistance without using any external exercise aids is a big part of isometric procedures. For example, by cupping your hands together and pulling to create tension, and holding that tension for several seconds at a time, you can help maintain a number of different upper body muscle systems.

Go to the library and check out a book about isometric exercise. You will learn a lot of commonsense approaches that can be applied during brief intervals throughout the workday.

Exercise possibilities are limitless.

To help your will power along, just ask yourself if you'd rather have your grandchildren push you around in a wheelchair once in a while at the care home, or be able to play hide and seek with them in your own home?

Choices. Choices.

You make them one way or another. Do you choose to do something, or to do nothing?

Your brain needs exercise, too

Physical exercise maintains strong muscle and bones as it creates movement of massive amounts of hormones, which are triggered by using our minds. That, in turn, creates much excitement amongst those neurons, which is hugely important in preventing such diseases as Parkinson's.

As children we enjoyed much physical activity, and created a lot of memories of pleasurable physical activity. Keep those memories alive by exciting them. Enjoy the physical activity you have enjoyed in the past. Participate in sports if that's your background, as there are activities and leagues for all ages.

Attend sporting events, whether it is your child's team or your favorite professional team. It will remind you of the time you made that touchdown that won the game fifty years ago.

If you want to double the positive hormone effect, take one of your children or an old sports teammate with you.

And if you're real brave, coach a team and knock down two birds with one stone. The physical activity, combined with memory stimulation, will help you build your defensive shield against AD even bigger.

Then when your team wins, the resulting testosterone surge will help steer you away from the advent of male menopause.

There is no greater feeling than that of being needed on an ongoing basis by twenty children. Someone has to pick up the slack created by more and more schools cutting out physical education. Frankly, the educational system has let down millions of children by depriving them of a very important factor in maintaining their health.

What good is intelligence if you can't maintain your health to use it?

If we would put physical education back into our schools, our children's cortisol levels would drop, along with ADHD, obesity, immune deficiencies, and illnesses caused by stress.

But then, that would be the logical thing to do. And logic is another commodity that has gone the way of the dodo bird along with common sense.

Chapter Fifteen: Key points to remember

Balancing yourself physically is as important as balancing your hormones, diet, and thought patterns.

There are many ways to get appropriate exercise.

Your brain needs exercise, too.

"If this country (America) is to survive, the best-fed nation myth had better be recognized for what it is, propaganda designed to produce wealth not health."

Adelle Davis

Chapter 16: Look for drug-free solutions

The biggest drug dealers in America sell their products legally. They are aided and abetted by doctors who prescribe those drugs to patients, who then make their buys at drug stores.

And the big drug company officers just keep on smiling as the money piles up into mountains of moola.

Even those TV ads that include the known side effects of the drugs being promoted have not slowed down the **Greed Express**.

How can that monster train be derailed?

It can be done, one railroad tie at a time, by health-conscious individuals who look for and find drug-free solutions.

Are you ready for this?

The biggest, best drug-free solution is food.

Use food as your drug

When consumed properly, food is a most powerful drug, and not just a form of pleasure as so many people think today. Those who consider that food was created as one of the purest forms of pleasure often are the same ones who can't see their feet until they sit down.

Doctors prescribe many drugs that actually exist within your body. Since this is so, doesn't it make sense to maintain proper levels of those internally manufactured drugs by the foods you eat?

Again, I can't recommend highly enough that you get Dr. Sears' book, *The Zone.* Also, his book*, Mastering The Zone.* Follow the food plans explained by Dr. Sears and you will be able to get and keep your body in balance.

Keep those good guys properly fed

A good, health-based diet will lay the foundation of building blocks needed for your body to produce its own drugs. This is something that you can control by eating properly.

Remember, think twice: weigh the immediate gratification with future consequences. A few moments of gluttony now, and possible disease later on; or, good food habits now which will make you soon feel better, and a larger defense shield against disease in the future?

Maintaining a 7-10 ratio of protein to carbohydrates is the best way to get the job done. As we discussed before, proteasomes are needed to grind up unwanted proteins such as beta amyloid, thereby helping to prevent AD.

Without the necessary building blocks made possible through proper diet, proteasomes just can't continue to be 100 percent defenders in your brain.

Make the weakest link stronger

There is a little saying out there: A chain is as strong as its weakest link. This holds true for amino acids, which are the building blocks of proteins.

For example, if you consume only 60 per cent of one of the eight essential amino acids you are going to inhibit all eight of them. And I would have to theorize that this deficiency would bring the effectiveness of proteasomes down to 60 per cent.

Drug manufacturers assure that they always have the products on hand to make their drugs.

Shouldn't you?

Like the drug manufacturers, you need to maintain supply of the building blocks at 100 percent to assure that the chain doesn't break.

And don't do it just once a day, but at every meal.

When was the last time you took a prescribed drug only once a day? You usually take them three times a day. Just like you should properly follow a health-based diet for optimum efficiency.

In regard to fats, you must consume them regularly to assure production of positive steroids, such as testosterone and estrogen, which are drugs produced by the body.

These are but two examples of the many drugs produced by the body.

We won't go into a discussion here; however, there are a wealth of different herbs, vitamins, and spices with which you can supplement your diet regimen to help assure that your body is better able to defend itself against disease.

In Chapter Two, the discussion of possible causes of AD included mention of aluminum. This metal can build up in your body, eventually posing a danger risk. A very natural way of getting aluminum out of your body is to take magnesium in supplement form. Aluminum binds to the magnesium, which is then eliminated through normal body processes, along with the aluminum that has bonded with it.

What is your answer to the following question?

The question I leave you with is this:

Do you want to eat a balanced diet, and help your body to be able to produce its own drugs, or do you want to eventually spend your life savings on expensive, unnatural substances from the legal drug dealers?

It's your choice.

Chapter Sixteen: Key points to remember

The biggest drug-free solution is food.

A balanced diet will help your body produce its own drugs.

Dr. Sears' books, *The Zone* and *Mastering The Zone*, can show you how to get tremendous drug-free benefits from food.

"A mind stretched by a new idea never goes back to its original dimension."

Oliver Wendell Holmes

Chapter 17: Reverse AD in early stages

Contrary to what the medical establishment would have you to believe, in its early stages, Alzheimer's Disease is quite reversible. It can be accomplished if both patient and doctor remove the barrier of denial. Don't just pass it off as being dementia.

If the mild symptoms, as outlined in Chapter One, are present, face up to the possibility that one is in the early stages of AD. Here is a re-listing of those symptoms:

Conscientiousness which declines

Vulnerability to stress which increases

Occasional depression

Loss of sense of smell

Knowledge is power. Once one's physical and mental status is determined, then, providing AD really is caught in its early stages, an effective plan of attack and defense can be put into motion.

The tools to get the job done are scattered throughout this book.

In some cases, people have reversed, or at least drastically slowed down the progression of AD, without really knowing that was what they were doing.

For example, the case of Willem de Kooning

Willem de Kooning (1904-1997) was a major figure in modern abstract expressionism. At about age 70 the artist began showing signs that his doctors diagnosed as AD.

He forgot people's names and recent events. To cover up his obvious confusion, he lied and made wisecracks. At times he would burst into rages; other times he lapsed into extended silences. He painted less and less until he stopped altogether.

Kooning's wife, Elaine, although separated from her husband for many years, did not accept the diagnosis. She re-entered de Kooning's life and aggressively led him through a series of lifestyle improvements. The four-step program that she implemented could have come straight out of this book, except that what she did took place nearly three decades ago.

Step One: He had been drinking so heavily that he suffered blackouts.
Solution: She got him to stop drinking.

Step Two: He had been eating poorly.
Solution: She got him on a healthy diet.

Step Three: He had become very sedentary.
Solution: She got him to exercise daily.

Step Four: He was sleeping irregularly.
Solution: She got him to sleep more.

Elaine's efforts paid off, as de Kooning regained mental sharpness and began painting again. His career continued for nearly ten years when he developed what his doctors called "true" AD.

I do not buy the notion that he was misdiagnosed previously. He was well into the AD progression, which was drastically slowed down through the efforts of a concerned and caring spouse.

Remember the power of love we discussed earlier?

Or the case of the bereaved widow

Let's call her Alma. At age 79, her husband died and she suffered progressive cognitive deterioration during the next six months. She was diagnosed as having AD.

The diagnosis came two months after she had sold their home and moved into a new condominium. In those new surroundings, during months five and six after her husband's death, Alma's AD symptoms progressed faster than is usually the case.

Investigation revealed that she had high blood levels of toluene, a toxic chemical used in construction materials. The toxicity apparently had accelerated the progression of AD.

Upon the advice of an environmental physician, Alma moved out of the condo, and into her daughter's older home. In just three weeks, Alma was back to her old self.

The combination of removing her from an environment that was toxic to her, and moving her to familiar surroundings with family, resulted in a reversal of AD symptoms.

Let's discuss these two cases.

Having his wife back in his life, de Kooning experienced pleasure again, and his immune system grew stronger, enabling his body to again produce its own drugs.

In effect, Elaine became her husband's personal doctor; however, a very wise one who knew that getting rid of the drugs (alcohol in this instance), and prescribing a regimen of proper diet, exercise, and sleep could only help.

The medicine of food helped restore some of the building blocks necessary so that his body could resume producing some of its own drugs.

The daily exercise helped to create positive hormonal movement and keep cortisol in check.

Proper sleep helped him to recover lost energy.

But, most important of all, was the reintroduction of pleasure through his wife's caring. This helped balance everything out.

Was an extra decade of productive painting and companionship with his wife worth it?

I think it was.

The widow's life was salvaged primarily through her move back into familiar surroundings. She went from being alone in a toxic, sterile environment to a home that no doubt had much pleasure and conversation daily.

Alma probably assisted in fixing the meals, which she made sure were properly balanced.

No longer did she just sit around worrying about where her next form of stimulation would come from to exercise those neurons to create excitement and stop cell degeneration. Her worries stopped and her cortisol levels went down.

The daughter had reversed roles, becoming doctor to her own mother. She gave back to Alma what Alma had once given to her, much love and needed attention.

Keep in mind that old adage

As the saying goes, "What comes around goes around." Take care of your children and they will take care of you.

Never has a family member of mine going back as far as five generations had AD. That's because there has never been a time when family members were denied places of pleasure in our homes or hearts.

We take care of our own.

No nursing homes or loneliness.

We sacrifice for our parents as they once sacrificed for us.

Remember, "What goes around comes around."

If you are not there for your children or spouse now, fulfilling their needs, they are not going to be around to fulfill your needs as you age.

Don't let your butt gather rust

Nip AD in the bud before it gets a chance to put down roots. At the first signs of depression, or when someone starts to become highly vulnerable to stress, those are often the first omens that AD is getting ready to kick in.

Do something about it. This book has armed you with effective fighting and defensive weapons. Use them. Don't be afraid to fire at the enemy. Better yet, use those tools before you have to dig a trench and hope that you have enough ammo left to force AD to retreat.

At least, do the basics:

Improve your diet.

Start to exercise.

Get a good night's sleep.

Seek positive pleasures in life.

And if your spouse or family is not there to help you with these endeavors, move on. There is no rule out there that says you can't fall in love again after age 50. If your children object, so what, it's your life and you have the right to enjoy it from birth until death.

Are you ready for this suggestion?

Should you not be interested in finding a mate, at least find ongoing companionship. There are many individuals out there in the same boat that you're in, just letting their lives sink away.

Speaking of boats, which are one of my hot buttons, why don't four of you get together and invest in a four-bedroom waterfront home with a dock and boat?

Let's see, depending on where you live, you can easily buy both for about $600,000. That's about $1,500 apiece if you get a thirty-year mortgage.

Before you start yelling about the expense, bear in mind that this represents about one-third the monthly cost of the average nursing home.

Use part of your savings to hire a full-time staff, and enjoy the rest of your life. You will probably be around to enjoy the pleasure of making the last payment for the second time in your life.

And when you finally kick the bucket, from old age and not AD, you will have something to pass on to your children or grandchildren, so they, too, can enjoy a most pleasurable retirement.

Chapter Seventeen: Key points to remember

In its early stages, Alzheimer's Disease is reversible.

Even in the case of someone diagnosed as having AD, like the example of the artist Willem de Kooning, it is possible for loving care and attention to enable one to reverse and drastically slow down the progression of symptoms. Kooning was able to enjoy more years of productive life because his wife didn't accept the doctors' diagnosis.

Kooning's wife assessed her husband's condition, and then did something to turn each negative into a positive.

The example of the bereaved widow shows that returning from a lonely environment to one in which the family shows loving care can reverse AD symptoms.

At the very least, do the basics:
Improve your diet.
Start to exercise.
Get a good night's sleep.
Seek positive pleasures in life.

"Judge a man by his questions rather than by his answers."

Voltaire

Chapter 18: Conflict of interest

"Who do you trust?"

That was a question asked years ago of contestants on a popular TV show.

Today, in what I call "the conflict of interest age," the question would be, "Who can I trust?"

Because it does not seem to me that there are many executives in the drug and medical industries that practice the time-honored Boy Scout specialty of being "trustworthy."

By "trustworthy," I mean always keeping the patients' and customers' best interests at heart.

What a challenge we face

For over three decades we've been herded down the path of depending on others to make our decisions for us. We have been told by our parents, and taught by our schools that we should let the experts make the decisions that control our lives.

After all, goes the argument, those experts know what is best for us.

But somewhere along the way, the concept of best interest became passé, with integrity getting trampled by the big boots of greed.

In far too many instances, best interest has given way to conflict of interest.

Common sense has been replaced by common cents that become dollars that become millions of dollars that become billions of dollars.

And who pays the tab, and suffers side effects that can and should be avoided?

For the most part, it is an unsuspecting public that has bought into the system, people who have bulls'-eyes on their wallets, and the drug and medical industries are out there target shooting.

Knowing what is going on is the first step toward facing up to the challenge that faces those of us who want fair-mindedness and integrity brought back to the forefront, especially in the drug and medical industries.

Along with getting an understanding of Alzheimer's in this book, you're getting a dose of truth that some people would prefer to keep buried under rock piles of subterfuge.

Until best interest takes priority, the number of AD victims will continue to increase.

A classic conflict of interest

The progression of events that led to FDA carte blanche approval for G.D. Searle to market aspartame as a food additive constituted a dramatic conflict of interest.

Aspartame, I believe, is by far the most dangerous of all food additives. This fact has been substantiated in numerous scientific studies that have been ignored by the Food and Drug Administration, which supposedly has the consumers' best interest at heart.

Aspartic acid (40%), phenylalanine (50%), and methanol (10%) comprise the substance called aspartame.

Methanol is commonly known as wood alcohol.

Isn't that considered a poison?

The Environmental Protection Agency (EPA) says so. They recommend limiting consumption to 7.8 mg per day. Yet a one-liter container of diet soda pop contains about 56 mg of methanol. Add to that the methanol contained in other products consumed containing aspartame, and you are well above the recommended limit.

We explained earlier what happens to wood alcohol when it is subjected to temperatures of 86 degrees F. and above.

Aspartame was discovered by accident in 1965 during testing of an anti-ulcer drug. And after much studying and testing, aspartame was approved for limited consumption in dry goods in July 1974.

However, approval was put on hold that year after the filing of an objection by neuroscientist Dr. John W. Olney and consumer attorney James Turner, who had disclosed to the FDA the true dangers of aspartame, along with the alleged devious research practices conducted by G.D. Searle.

An FDA staff majority voiced fears of aspartame dangers should the product be approved for consumption with food and beverages. It took the replacement of the FDA commissioner by President Ronald Reagan to make way for such approval, which came for use as a food additive in 1981, and later, 1983, for inclusion with beverages.

Soon after gaining the much sought after approval, the FDA commissioner became dean of a New York medical college, then was hired as a consultant with G.D. Searle's public relations firm, Burson-Marstellar, at a reported $1,000 a day.

Is it mere coincidence that the rapid rise in AD cases has paralleled the proliferation of aspartame into thousands of food and beverage products?

What do you think?

A revolving door of greed

I won't belabor the issue here; however, some "watch-dog" agencies in Washington, D.C. have high turnover rates among upper staff positions. A lot of those folks wind up on the payrolls of companies for whom they engineered favorable decisions.

That is the ultimate conflict of interest.

It's like a revolving door of greed.

Which raises the question, "Exactly who is doing the research or reviewing submitted research to protect our best interests?

It's not the FDA, that's for sure.

The November, 1992 Townsend Letter for Doctors reported on a study revealing that 37 of 49 FDA high-level officers who left the FDA took well-paying positions with companies they had regulated. The report also indicated that over 150 FDA officials owned stock in drug companies they were assigned to monitor.

In May 2000 the FDA re-approved NutraSweet.

Only recently, after banning it for many years, did the FDA approve the natural sweetener stevia to be sold in the United States, and then only as a supplement and not as food.

Could it be that this perfectly natural and safe product might develop into competition for aspartame?

On a level playing field where one's best interests are championed, it certainly would be possible. A huge percentage of Japan's population chooses to use stevia as an alternative sweetener. Doesn't that make you wonder what the Japanese know that we don't know?

A caution about side effects

I've preached to you hard about doing what it takes to get and keep your brain and body in proper balance via the big four of diet, exercise, sleep, and pleasure.

Drug-free solutions, I believe, are always best if possible to pursue, in part because they allow you to avoid a wide range of side effects caused by ingesting drugs.

When considering any medication, read the label on the container, especially the small print. Ask yourself if this new drug or additive is going to conflict with your balance. If so, how much?

If the label says headache, you know the product is going to have an effect on your mind.

That is just common sense.

If it says that your liver will have to be monitored, beware, because that product will take you out of balance. Your liver is so important in removing toxins that get into your body from environmental causes and through the food and beverages that you consume. Mess with that filtering capability so that it slows or shuts down liver function, and toxins will build up in your brain.

Try asking your doctor or pharmacist what the side effects are for a particular drug that you've been recommended to take, and you'll likely run into a wall of silence.

Then into your hands will be placed one of those colorful brochures published by the drug manufacturer. On the cover is this beautiful setting, and a smiling individual. And as you flip through it, the language quickly turns into Greek and as you continue the print gets so small that you can't even read it. That's where you will find the listing of side effects.

Listen to the rapid reciting of side effects the next time you see a TV commercial pitching how wonderful a particular drug is. It's like describing Dr. Jeckyl and Mr. Hyde in one breath. And the pitch person does it with a straight face.

An interesting poll

A year 2000 poll conducted over the Internet by The Alzheimer's Association asked this question: "Do you think the government is doing enough to support Alzheimer research?"

Of 5,121 respondents, 92.7% (4,746) voted No, while only 7.3% (375) voted Yes.

Actually, the best thing that could happen in D.C. is for the many regulatory agencies, the FDA for example, to simply perform their specified duties in an unbiased manner, which really would be in our best interest.

What a novel thought.

One of the benefits that would accrue to the government would be at least the perceived notion that it was in favor of all manner of research in regard to disease in general.

I'd like to see some form of research funding that comes directly from the public, you and me. Not from big business or the government, as that always comes with strings attached.

How could this be done?

Well, here's an idea for starters. You might have a better idea. If so, I'd like to hear about it. Meanwhile, consider this possibility:

Add $10 to your next tax return. Request in writing that you want the IRS to set the money aside in a special, restricted account to be used so that we, the public, can create an organization funded solely by us. Said organization to conduct research as to the cause of disease so preventative means, rather than just more drug development, can be implemented.

Heck, make it interesting for the IRS. Send $15: $10 for research, $2 for IRS administrative costs, and $3 to donate to any politician who will support our true best interests.

OK, OK. So you think it's an outlandish idea. At least it's an idea. How do you think it could be done?

Meanwhile, by participating in the questionnaire in the next chapter, you can help advance AD research that truly is unbiased.

Chapter Eighteen: Key points to remember

Conflicts of interest that influence government officials, government agency officials, major manufacturers, the drug and medical industries, drastically affect the quality of healthcare in the United States.

A classic conflict of interest is illustrated by the history of how aspartame came to be approved by the FDA.

Be wary of any product that can induce side effects when ingested.

Participate in the questionnaire in the next chapter. By doing so, you will help advance AD research that really is unbiased.
****

"The value of an idea lies in the using of it."

Thomas Edison

Chapter 19: Taking control of our destinies

Thomas Edison hit the nail solidly on the head with that statement. And that principle holds just as true with the many commonsense methods of preventing AD that I've presented to you in this book.

But what good will any of these ideas do if you don't use them?

All of the proposed methods are safer than any prescribed drug, in that none of them have any known negative side effects whatsoever.

And the methods are supported with facts coming out of ideal study conditions (real life). Such facts do not lie as they are etched in history.

Some of the methods are optional depending upon your age; however, if you are a parent with young children, the suggested methods are much more an obligation than an option. Take control of your children's destiny until they are old enough to leave home and take over the reins of their own futures.

Now for the questionnaire

As you've made it this far in the book, you know the tremendous good that can happen with thousands and thousands of people randomly answering the questions in the questionnaire.

Massive participation could mark a major turning point in AD research, as causes will be pinpointed, which can lead to prevention rather then just treating symptoms with drugs.

The bottom line is that research developed from processing many thousands of respondents' answers will enable more people to avoid AD and live long, productive, enjoyable lives.

Whether you've ordered this book in trade paperback or electronic format from our web site, please go to our site now – http://www.lodgecreekresearch.com – and click on the "Questionnaire" icon. Read the instructions, and then answer the questions. As soon as you've finished, click on "All Done." Your completed questionnaire will instantly enter processing.

Following are the preliminary questions that precede the actual questionnaire, followed by the questionnaire.

Thank you in advance for helping advance commonsense research that is unbiased with no strings attached.

QUESTIONNAIRE

Preliminary questions:

Age_____
Sex:
a. male
b. female
Alzheimer's Disease:
a. yes
b. no
If yes:
a. late onset
b. early onset
c. familiar
d. sporadic
e. Age of onset_____
Gene type:
a. ApoE-4/ApoE-4
b. ApoE-4/ApoE-3
c. ApoE-4/ApoE-2
d. ApoE-3/ApoE-3
e. ApoE-3/ApoE-2
f. ApoE-2/ApoE-2

g. Unknown

Dementias, other than Alzheimer's:

a. yes

b. no

If yes:

What age? _____

If yes:

Have you recovered?

a. yes

b. no

Arthritis:

a. yes

b. no

If yes, method of treatment:

a. physical exercise

b. nonsteroid anti-inflammatory drugs

c. cortisteroid

d. none

Parkinson's Disease:

a. yes

b. no

If yes:

a. late onset

b. early onset

c. familiar

d. sporadic

If yes, related to A.D.:

a. yes

b. no

Other health problems:

a. diabetes

b. arteriosclerosis

c. head injury

d. obesity

e. depression

f. other _____

Menopause:
a. yes
b. no
c. unknown
If yes:
What age? _____
If yes:
Estrogen replacement therapy?
a. yes
b. no
How many children do you have? _____
Your age when the last child left home: _____
As a child were you:
a. naturally breast fed
b. fed breast milk through bottle
c. formula
d. other _____

Here are the one hundred questions:

Prenatal

1. Mother's stress level during pregnancy:
   a. None   b. Low
   c. Moderate   d. High
   e. Unknown
2. Mother's diet during pregnancy:
   a. Balanced   b. High carbohydrate
   c. High protein d. Vegetarian
   e. Unknown
3. Mother's alcohol consumption during pregnancy:
   a. None   b. 1-2 times a month
   c. 1-2 times a week   d. 1-2 times a day
   e. More they 2 per day   f. Unknown
   Product consumed:

   a. Beer   b. Wine
   c. Liquor
4. Mother's illegal drug consumption during pregnancy:
   a. None   b. Low
   c. Moderate   d. High
5. Mother's marital status during pregnancy:
   a. Single   b. Married
   c. Divorced   d. Widowed

Birth to Age 2

6. Parental daily contact:
   a. None   b. 1-3 hours a day
   c. 3 -5 hours a day   d. 6 hours or more a day
   e. Less then 1 Hour   f. Unknown
7. Contact with relatives:
   a. None   b. Daily
   c. Weekly   d. Monthly
   e. Yearly
8. Parent's marital status:
   a. Single   b. Married
   c. Divorced   d. Widowed
9. Location:
   a. Rural   b. Urban
   c. Suburban   d. Big city
10. Daycare:
   a. Stay home Mom   b. Daycare Center
   c. Relative care   d. Nanny (live in)

Age 2 to 5

11. Parents' marital status:
   a. Single   b. Married
   c. Divorced   d. Widowed
12. Parental daily contact:
   a. None   b. 1-3 hours a day

c. 3-5 hours a day   d. 6 hours or more a day
e. Less they 1 hour   f. Unknown

13. Contact with relatives during this age:
   a. None   b. Daily
   c. Weekly   d. Monthly
   e. Yearly

14. Location:
   a. Rural   b. Urban
   c. Suburban   d. Big city

15. Daycare:
   a. Stay home Mom   b. Daycare Center
   c. Relative care   d. Nanny (live in)

16. Diet:
   a. Balanced   b. High carbohydrates
   c. High protein   d. Vegetarian

17. Exposure to traumatic experience:
   a. Abandonment   b. Sexual abuse
   c. Physical abuse   d. Violent act
   e. None

18. Exposure to positive nurturing in general:
   a. None   b. Low
   c. Moderate   d. High

19. Stress levels:
   a. None   b. Low
   c. Moderate   d. High

20. Environment in general:
   a. Nurturing   b. Non-nurturing
   c. Stressful   d. Abusive

Age 5 to 12

21. Parents' marital status:
   a. Single   b. Married
   c. Divorced   d. Widowed

22. Parental daily contact:
   a. None   b. 1-3 hours a day

c. 3-5 hours a day　　d. 6 hours or more a day
e. Less then 1 Hour　　f. Unknown

23. Contact with relatives during this age:
　a. None　　　　　　b. Daily
　c. Weekly　　　　　d. Monthly
　e. Yearly

24. Location:
　a. Rural　　　　　　b. Urban
　c. Suburban　　　　d. Big city

25. Schooling
　a. Public　　　　　b. Private
　c. Home　　　　　　d. None

26. Diet:
　a. Balanced　　　　b. High carbohydrates
　c. High protein　　d. Vegetarian

27. Exposure to traumatic experience:
　a. Abandonment　　b. Sexual abuse
　c. Physical abuse　d. Violent act
　d. None

28. Exposure to positive nurturing in general:
　a. None　　　　　　b. Low
　c. Moderate　　　　d. High

29. Stress levels:
　a. None　　　　　　b. Low
　c. Moderate　　　　d. High

30. Environment in general:
　a. Nurturing　　　　b. Non-nurturing
　c. Stressful　　　　d. Abusive

Age 12 to 18

31. Parents' marital status:
　a. Single　　　　　b. Married
　c. Divorced　　　　d. Widowed

32. Parental daily contact:
　a. None　　　　　　b. 1-3 hours a day

    c. 3-5 hours a day   d. 6 hours or more a day
    e. Unknown
33. Contact with relatives during this age:
    a. None   b. Daily
    c. Weekly   d. Monthly
    e. Yearly
34. Location:
    a. Rural   b. Urban
    c. Suburban   d. Big city
35. Schooling
    a. Public   b. Private
    c. Home   d. None
36. Diet:
    a. Balanced   b. High carbohydrates
    c. High protein   d. Vegetarian
37. Exposure to traumatic experience:
    a. Abandonment   b. Sexual abuse
    c. Physical abuse   d. Violent act
    e. None
38. Exposure to positive nurturing in general:
    a. None   b. Low
    c. Moderate   d. High
39. Stress levels:
    a. None   b. Low
    c. Moderate   d. High
40. Environment in general:
    a. Nurturing   b. Non-nurturing
    c. Stressful   d. Abusive

Childhood in General

41. Education level:
    a. Grades 1-6   b. Grades 6-9
    c. Grades 9-12   d. None
42. Physical activity:
    a. Low   b. Moderate
    c. High   d. None
43. Number of siblings in household:
    a. 1   b. 2
    c. 3   d. 4
    e. 5-7   f. 8-10
    g. 10 or more
44. Exposure to toxins:
    a. Pesticides and herbicides
    b. Industrial toxins through water
    c. Occupational Exposure
    d. Industrial toxins through air
    e. None
45. General attitude:
    a. Optimistic   b. Pessimistic
46. Parental guidance in general:
    a. Low   b. Moderate
    c. High   d. None
47. Family's average financial status through childhood:
    a. Poverty   b. Below average
    c. Average   d. Above average
48. Long-term childhood friendships:
    a. 0 to 2   b. 2 to 4
    c. 4 to 6   d. 6 or more
49. Family type:
    a. Traditional family b. Single parent family
    c. Foster family   d. Adoptive family
50. General health:
    a. Poor   b. Fair
    c. Good   d. Excellent

Age 18 to 25

51. College education:
    a. 1-2 years   b. 3-4 years
    c. Graduate school   d. None
52. Diet:
    a. Balanced   b. High carbohydrates
    c. High protein   d. Vegetarian
53. Physical activity:
    a. Low   b. Moderate
    c. High   d. None
54. Stress levels:
    a. None   b. Low
    c. Moderate   d. High
55. Location:
    a. Rural   b. Urban
    c. Suburban   d. Big city
56. Contact with relatives during this age:
    a. None   b. Daily
    c. Weekly   d. Monthly
    e. Yearly
57. Parental contact:
    a. None   b. Daily
    c. Weekly   d. Monthly
    e. Yearly
58. Marital status
    a. Single   b. Married
    c. Divorced   d. Widowed
59. Consumption of alcohol:
    a. None   b. 1-2 times a month
    c. 1-2 times a week   d. 1-2 times a day
    e. More then 2 per day
    Product consumed:
    a. Beer
    b. Wine
    c. Liquor

60. Personal interests carried over from childhood:
   a. None   b. Few
   c. Some   d. Many

Age 25 to 40

61. Continuing education:
   a. 1 year or less   b. 2-3 years
   c. 4 or more years   d. None
62. Diet:
   a. Balanced   b. High carbohydrates
   c. High protein   d. Vegetarian
63. Physical activity:
   a. Low   b. Moderate
   c. High   d. None
64. Stress levels:
   a. None   b. Low
   c. Moderate   d. High
65. Location:
   a. Rural   b. Urban
   c. Suburban   d. Big city
66. Contact with relatives during this age:
   a. None   b. Daily
   c. Weekly   d. Monthly
   e. Yearly
67. Parental contact:
   a. None   b. Daily
   c. Weekly   d. Monthly
   e. Yearly
68. Marital status
   a. Single   b. Married
   c. Divorced   d. Widowed
69. Consumption of alcohol:
   a. None   b. 1-2 times a month
   c. 1-2 times a week   d. 1-2 times a day
   e. More then 2 per day

Product consumed:
  a. Beer
  b. Wine
  c. Liquor
70. Personal interests carried over from childhood:
  a. None   b. Few
  c. Some   d. Many

Age 40 to 60

71. Continuing education:
  a. 1 year or less   b. 2-3 years
  c. 4 or more years   d. None
72. Diet:
  a. Balanced   b. High carbohydrates
  c. High protein   d. Vegetarian
73. Physical activity:
  a. Low   b. Moderate
  c. High   d. None
74. Stress levels:
  a. None   b. Low
  c. Moderate   d. High
75. Location:
  a. Rural   b. Urban
  c. Suburban   d. Big city
76. Contact with relatives during this age:
  a. None   b. Daily
  c. Weekly   d. Monthly
  e. Yearly
77. Parental contact:
  a. None   b. Daily
  c. Weekly   d. Monthly
  e. Yearly
78. Marital status:
  a. Single   b. Married
  c. Divorced   d. Widowed

79. Consumption of alcohol:
   a. None   b. 1-2 times a month
   c. 1-2 times a week   d. 1-2 times a day
   e. More then 2 per day
 Product consumed:
   a. Beer
   b. Wine
   c. Liquor
80. Personal interests carried over from childhood:
   a. None   b. Few
   c. Some   d. Many

Age 60 and Over

81. Retirement activities: Age of retirement _____
   a. Volunteering   b. Continuing occupation
   c. Music   d. Gardening
   e. Travel   f. None
82. Diet:
   a. Balanced   b. High carbohydrates
   c. High protein   d. Vegetarian
83. Physical activity:
   a. Low   b. Moderate
   c. High   d. None
84. Stress levels:
   a. None   b. Low
   c. Moderate   d. High
85. Location:
   a. Rural   b. Urban
   c. Suburban   d. Big city
86. Contact with relatives during this age:
   a. None   b. Daily
   c. Weekly   d. Monthly
   e. Yearly
87. Parental contact:
   a. None   b. Daily

   c. Weekly   d. Monthly
   e. Yearly

88. Marital status
   a. Single   b. Married
   c. Divorced   d. Widowed

89. Consumption of alcohol:
   a. None   b. 1-2 times a month
   c. 1-2 times a week   d. 1-2 times a day
   e. More then 2 per day

Product consumed:
   a. Beer
   b. Wine
   c. Liquor

90. Personal interests carried over from childhood:
   a. None   b. Few
   c. Some   d. Many

Adulthood in General

91. Stress in General:
   a. None   b. Low
   c. Moderate   d. High

92. Pleasure in General:
   a. None   b. Low
   c. Moderate   d. High

93. Marital enjoyment:
   a. None   b. Low
   c. Moderate   d. High

94. Family involvement:
   a. None   b. Low
   c. Moderate   d. High

95. Consumption of aspartame:
   a. 1-2 products per day
   b. 2-4 products per day
   c. 4-6 products per day
   d. 6 or more products per day

e. None
96. Ongoing close friendly relationships:
   a. None   b. 1-2 friends
   c. 3-4 friends   d. 4 or more
97. Financial status through adulthood:
   a. $20,000 or less year
   b. $20,000 to $40,000 per year
   c. $40,000 to $60,000 per year
   d. $60,000 to $100,000 per year
   e. $100,000 to $150,000 per year
   f. $150,000 or more

98. Family type:
   a. Traditional family   b. Single parent family
   c. Foster family   d. Adoptive family
99. General Health through adulthood:
   a. Poor   b. Fair
   c. Good   d. Excellent
100. Would you consider supporting unbiased publicly funded
   preventative research?
   a. YES   b. NO

Chapter Nineteen: Key points to remember

None of the commonsense methods presented in this book have any negative side effects.

By participating in the questionnaire, you have helped advance the cause of unbiased AD research.

Chapter Resources

Chapter 1

10 Warning Signs of Early Alzheimer's Disease
http://www.alzheimers.com/health_library/diagnosis/diagnosis
_02_warning.html

Book: "The Brain Encyclopedia" Copyright 1996
by Carol Turkington

Alzheimer's Disease - Unraveling the Mystery (Aug. 1995)
http://www.alzheimers.org/unravel.html

Areas of Research Focus
http://www.alzheimers.uci.edu/research.html

Chapter 2

Researchers restart brain cell growth (Associated Press)
http://www.msnbc.com/news/326588.asp

MGH Researchers Connect Alzheimer's Mutations to Cell
Death Process
Doctors Guide to Medical & other news
http//www.docguide.com.nsf/ge/unregistered.user.545434

Depression May Be An Early Sign of Alzheimer's Disease
Alzheimers.com Newsroom (12/9/99)
*http://www.alzheimers.com/news/index.html

Stress & Your Brain
By: John D. MacArthur
Brain.com
http://www.brain.com/about/article.cfm?id=2082&cat_id=39

Flouride Fact Sheet
http://www.earthlife.org.za/factsheets/fs_flouride.htm

The Bitter Truth About Artificial Sweeteners
http://www.nexusmagazine.com/Aspartame.html

Suppression of emotion impairs memory New York (July 26, 1999)
Brain.com
http://www.brain.com/about/article.cfm?id=2187&cat_id=35

Poor Childhood Nutrition Linked to Alzheimer's
Alzheimers.com Newsroom (Nov. 9 1998)
*http://www.alzheimers.com

Chapter 3

Book: "Inside The Brain" Copyright 1996,1997 by Ronald Kotulak and
The Chicago Tribune

What's Going On In There? How the Brain and Mind Develop in the First Five
Brain.com
http://www.brain.com/about/article.cfm?id=2421&cat_id=61

Large Families May Induce Alzheimer's
http://abcnews.go.com/sections/living/DailyNews/Alzheimers_00126.html

Chapter 4

The Amazing Power of Support Groups
http://www.alzheimers.com/health_library/coping/coping_12_support.html

Married People Less Likely To Develop Alzheimer's
Alzheimers.com Newsroom (12/30/99)
http://www.alzheimers.com/news/1991230-2527.html

AARP Modern Maturity, July-August 00
The Allure of Money
By Susan Jacoby

Happy Times May Not Reduce Stress Hormones in Some People
(Aug. 4, 2000) (Reuters)
http://www.brain.com/about/article.cfm?id=15102&cat_id=39

Lack of Sleep Alters Hormones, Metabolism
Oct. 22, 1999
http://www.pslgroup.com/dg/13d2f2.htm

Happy Times May Not Reduce Stress Hormones in Some People
Aug. 4, 2000 (Reuters)
http://www.brain.com/about/article.cfm?id=15102&at_ID=39

Chapter 5

Happy times may reduce stress hormones in some people
Aug 04' 2000 (Reuter)
http://www.brain.com/about/article.cfm?ID=15102&cat_ID=3
9

My Love Is Chemical
By: James Adam
*http://www.brain.com/about/full_list_article.cfm?id=35

The Quest For Aphrodesia
By: John D. MacArthur
http://www.brain.com/about/article.cfm?id=6504&cat_id=37

Book: "Inside The Brain" Copyright 1996-1997
By: Ronald Kotulak and The Chicago Tribune

Chapter 6

Yahoo News
Health Headlines
Friday, Jan. 28, 6:09 p.m. EST
Music Therapy Helps Alzheimer's Patients
By: Jane Vail

Chapter 7

Retirement statistics: U.S. Bureau of Vital Statistics, 1980, 1990

Chapter 8

U.S. News: Inside the Teen Brain: Young Minds Are Still Taking Shape
(8/9/99)
By: Shannon Brownlee
http://www.usnews.com/usnews/issue/990809/nycu/teenbrain.htm

Press Release: Wednesday April 7, 1999, 2 p.m. EST
Brigham and Women's Research Team Identifies Enzyme that Initiates Alzheimer's Disease

Chicago Tribune Archives - Theory Links Brain's Repair System To Alzheimer's.
Nu Scientist believes Evolutionary Flaw is Key To Deciphering Disease
By: Ronald Kotulak, Tribune Staff/ Sun. Dec. 19, 1999

Chapter 9

Testosterone May Reduce Production of Alzheimer's Protein
Alzheimers.com Newsroom (1/31/00)
http://www.alzheimers.com/news/20000131-3023.html

The Role of Melatonin and Serotonin in Aging: Update
By: B.R. Grady & R. Rozencwaig
wysiwyg://66/http://www.mediconsult.com/m...onin/journal/au
tomation/960102017001.html

Male Menopause - fact or fiction?
By: Dr. Malcom Carruthers, MD, FRCPath, MRCGP
Home Page - Gold Cross Medical Services

Memory - Stress & Your Brain
By: John D. MacArthur
http://www.brain.com/about/article.cfm?id=2082&cat_id=39

Book: "Enter The Zone" by Barry Sears, Ph.D. w/ Bill Lawren

Chapter 10

Alzheimer's Risk Factor Explained
By: Penny Stern, MD - Alzheimers.com
http://www.alzheimers.com/news/2000302-3481.html

Unraveling the Mystery - A.D. - (Aug. 1995)
http://www.alzheimers.org/unravel.html

Genetic Lifestyle Factors Contribute to Dimentia Risk
Alzheimers.com Newsroom (7/9/99)
http://www.alzheimers.com/news/19990709-01.html

Mitochondria Gene Defects Linked to Alzheimer's Disease
By: Keith Mulvihill

Alzheimers.com Newsroom (Sep.4 00)
http://www.alzheimers.com/news/20000720-6747.html

Doctors Guide – It's Not Just What You Eat That Affects Risk
For Heart Disease & Stroke
http//www.docguide.com.nsf/ge/unregistered.user.545434

New Clues to Alzheimer's Disease
By: Penny Stern, M.D.
Alzheimers.com
http://www.alzheimers.com/news/20000404-4087.html

Alzheimer's Risk Factor Explained
An Unexpected Trust in Alzheimer's Research
By: Holly Weng
(1994, Vertices 10 (1):23-24

Proteasomes Break Down Unneeded Proteins
http://www.abc.net.au/science/news/stories/S51747.html

Mitochondria Gene Defects Linked To Alzheimer's Disease
By: Keith Mulvihill
Alzheimers.com Newsroom Sept. 4, 00
http://www.alzheimers.com/news/20000720-6747.html

Atlas of Protein Side-Chain Interactions
http://www.biochem.ucl.ac.uk/csm/sidechains/

Fat
http://health.aol.drkoop.com/conditions/ency/article/002468.ht
ml

Fats In Nutrition
By: Ron Kennedy, M.D. Santa Rosa, California
http://www.medical-library.net/sites/_fats_in_nutrition.html

Chapter 11

Proteins in Nutrition
By: Ron Kennedy, M.D. Santa Rosa, California
http://www.medical-library.net/sites_proteins_in_nutrition.html

The Macronutrients
By: Ron Kennedy, M.D. Santa Rosa, California
http://www.medical-library.net/sites/_macronutrients_(whole_food).html

Eicosanoid Balance and Essential Fatty Acids
By: Ron Kennedy, M.D. Santa Rosa, California
http://www.medical-library.net/sites/_eicosanoid_balance_and_essential_fatty_acids.html

Protein/Nutrition Center
http://www.health.aol.drkoop.com/wellness/nutrition/vitamins_minerals/index.asp?id=25

Nutritional Deficiency Dementia (Diagnosis)
http://www.alzheimers.com/health_library/diagnosis/diagnosis_12_nutri.html

Fat Increases the Risk of Alzheimer's Disease
http://www.brain.com/about/article.cfm?id=14000&cat_id=16

Chapter 12

Article - Lighten Up
Dynamics Online (1998)

Neuroscience for Kids - Laughter and the Brain
http://weber.u.washington.edu/~chudler/laugh.html

Laughter Brings Us Happiness
http://www.ic-net.or.jp/home/tsato/page2-2html

Laughter Is Good For You
http://www.makeemlaugh.com/science.html

How to be Funnier - Healthwise Humor
http://www.sprintout.com/funnybook/health.html

An Apple A Day
It's Laughter We're After
By: Jenny Herrick, RN, BAS - Humor Program Mgr.
St. Lukes Regional Medical Center
http://www.siouxlan.com/stlukes/HLHUM7.html

Stress and Your Brain
By: John D. MacArthur
http://www.brain.com/about/articlecfm?id=2082&cat_id=39

Stress Causes Illnesses
By: Sarah Wight The Murray State News
http://www.thenews.org/02287/stress.html

Poor Childhood Nutrition Linked to Alzheimer's
Alzheimers.com Newsroom (Nov. 9, 1998)
http://www.Alzheimers_com/news/19981109-01.html

Book: "Enter The Zone" Copyright 1995 by: Barry Sears, Ph.D. w/ Bill Lawren

Carbohydrates in Nutrition
By: Ron Kennedy, M.D., Santa Rosa, California
http://www.medical.library.net/sites/_carbohydrates_in_nutrition.html

Chapter 13

Love on the Brain: A Review of "A General Theory of Love"
By: Sarah Koenig
http://www.brain.com/about/article.cfm?ID=9100&cat_ID=40
0

Book: "Inside the Brain" Copyright 1996-1997
by: Ronald Kotulak and The Chicago Tribune

Stressful Job May be Hazardous to Health
(May 26, 2000) Reuters
http://www.brain.com/about/article/cfm?id=1171&cat_id=39

Chapter 14

Cope w/ Stress / Alzheimers.com
http://www.alzheimers.com/health_library/coping/coping_13_s
tress.html

Book: "The Feeling Good Handbook" Copyright 1989
by: David D. Burns, M. D.

Chapter 15

New Stress Management Program Increases DHEA and
Reduces Cortisol Levels
http://www.heartmath.org/ro/hro/hemo3.html

Doctors Guide
AAN Meeting: Regular Physical Activity May Protect Against
Alzheimer's Disease
http//www.docguide.com.nsf/ge/unregistered.user.545434

Stress and Your Brain
By: John D. MacArthur

http:/www.brain.com/about/articlecfm?id=2082&cat_id=39

Chapter 16

Book: "Enter the Zone" Copyright 1995
By: Barry Sears, Ph.D. w/ Bill Lawren

Proteasomes Break Down Unneeded Proteins
http://www.abc.net.au/science/news/stories/S51747.html

Atlas of Protein Side-Chain Interactions
http://www.biochem.uc/.ac.uk/bsm/sidechains/

Proteins in Nutrition
By: Ron Kennedy, M.D. Santa Rosa, California
http://www.medical.library.net/sites/_proteins_in_nutrition.htm

Parkinsons Gene Discovery May Implicate Brain's Protein
Disposal System In Other Neurodegenerative Diseases
National Institutes of Health
http://www.brain.com/about/article.cfm?10=534&cat_10=4

Chapter 17

How to Stay Mentally Sharp – For Life, Part II
Alzheimers.com (Risk Factors & Prevention)
http://www.alzheimers.com/health_library/risk/risk_05_sharp2
html

Other Causes of Dementia – Overview
Alzheimers.com (Diagnosis)
http://www.alzheimers.com/health_library/diagnosis/diagnosis
_07_dimentias.htm

Atlas of Protein Side-Chain Interactions
http://www.biochem.ucl.uc.uk/bsm/sidechains/

Chapter 18

Aspartame… The Bad News!
http://www.dorway.com/badnews.html
Article Courtesy of Mark Gold @ mgold@tiac.net

Debunking the "Official Aspartame Myth"
(Aug. 1992)
What You Should Know About Aspartame
http://www.dorway.com/offaspart.html

Aspartame's Sordid History To Market With References
http://www.dorway.com/enclosur.html
Alzheimer's Association Previous Poll Results
http://www.alz.org/previouspoll.html

Sightings: Read The Deadly Truth About Aspartame (NutraSweet, Equal, Spoonful, etc.)
By: Nancy Marlle
12/12/98
http://www.sightings.com/health/sweetners.html

About the author

James F. Watson is unique in the world of Alzheimer's research. When his wife Sandy began exhibiting symptoms of Alzheimer's Disease, he devoted his life to discovering – for himself, independently of mainstream AD research – the many causes of AD.

During several years of intense effort, Watson began applying what he had discovered toward the goal of reversing Sandy's AD symptoms.

Upon achieving that incredible goal, Watson felt he must share his findings with others.

Commonsense Approaches to Alzheimer's was birthed.

CPSIA information can be obtained at www.ICGtesting.com

233508LV00007B/18/P